DARE TO TRI

My Journey from the BBC Breakfast Sofa to GB Team Triathlete

LOUISE MINCHIN

BLOOMSBURY SPORT

LONDON · OXFORD · NEW YORK · NEW DELHI · SYDNEY

BLOOMSBURY SPORT
Bloomsbury Publishing Plc
50 Bedford Square, London, WC1B 3DP, UK

BLOOMSBURY, BLOOMSBURY SPORT and the Diana logo are trademarks of
Bloomsbury Publishing Plc

First published in Great Britain 2018

A catalogue record for this book is available from the British Library

Library of Congress Cataloguing-in-Publication data has been applied for

ISBN: PB: 978-1-4729-4918-9; eBook: 978-1-4729-4917-2

2 4 6 8 10 9 7 5 3 1

Typeset in ITC Century by Deanta Global Publishing Services, Chennai, India
Printed and bound in Great Britain by CPI Group (UK) Ltd. Croydon, CRO 4YY

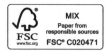

MIX
Paper from
responsible sources
FSC
www.fsc.org   FSC® C020471

To find out more about our authors and books visit www.bloomsbury.com
and sign up for our newsletters

I would like to dedicate this book to David, Mia and Scarlett, my wonderful husband and daughters. Without your love, support and patience, I couldn't have been on this incredible journey. Thank you for making it possible, and for being part of it, and supporting me every step of the way.

CONTENTS

FOREWORD BY DAME DARCEY BUSSELL

Louise's amazing journey to becoming a triathlete encourages us all to be a little more adventurous.

I think (!) she won't mind me writing this, but it is precisely because Louise is *not* an overly exceptional athlete that her wonderful personal achievements are so encouraging. In fact, I remember many times being on holiday with her when the most energetic things she did all week were swim just a little, read a book and sunbathe.

This all changed, though, once she took up triathlon at the age of 45.

Louise made this decision despite being a full-time working mother who juggles the responsibilities of family, work, dogs, a very old cat (which I have tripped over numerous times in her kitchen), several rabbits, miniature ponies that regularly escape and her exceptionally early 3:30 a.m. starts.

In Louise's endeavour to compete for Great Britain in triathlon, she made use of attributes that we all actually possess, especially if we dig a little: bravery, mental strength and determination. She used them brilliantly – and to the full!

Being a bit stubborn and a little competitive, Louise saw the opportunity to make the British team in her age division, and took it. As you can imagine, this was an adventure not without its incidents, as Louise faced fear, danger and disappointment, as well as success.

By her example, she shows us that we should strive to be our best and to grab opportunities that are offered to us – or forge them ourselves if they are not immediately obvious, finding both the courage and determination to do so.

Dare to Tri reminds us that we all have different strengths, that we are never too old to start a new challenge and that life is wonderful.

As Louise strove to become a British athlete, she found a strength that she did not think she possessed, embraced a new outlook on life and fitness – and she never ever gave up, one of her finest qualities.

Well done, my old friend!

Darcey x

INTRODUCTION

Five years ago, if anyone had suggested to me that there was the slightest possibility I could compete in a triathlon and represent my country, I would have told them to stop being ridiculous. What an absurd thing to say!

I didn't even know quite what a triathlon was. I had an inkling it involved swimming, running and cycling. I knew that a pair of brothers from Yorkshire were very good at it. But what did you do first – swim, run, or cycle? How did you change from one sport to the other? And how far did you have to race? I had no idea.

Apart from being clueless, I wasn't even looking for a sporting challenge, and I certainly didn't class myself as an athlete or particularly sporty.

I was a long-term resident of the *BBC Breakfast* sofa, a working Mum in her mid-40s who had given up competitive sport as a teenager. The only exercise I did was to occasionally ride my bike a few miles into work. Being involved in an endurance sport and representing my country was unthinkable – completely beyond my imagination.

So, what changed? How did I get from a fun *BBC Breakfast* Christmas Challenge to daring to think that I could represent my country?

This book tells the story of how I discovered a sport that became a passion and then an obsession. It describes an adventure that has not been without its challenges. I have struggled along the way, overcoming nerves, personal disappointment and the odd bike crash.

My triathlon journey has tested me to the limit mentally and physically, an experience both unexpected and exhilarating. It has made me fitter, stronger, happier, and awoken in me a competitive spirit and a love of sport that I assumed I had lost.

Here is my story.

Louise x

CHAPTER 1

THE START OF THE ADVENTURE

'The most exhilarating, satisfying and memorable half-second of my life.'

The moment I touched the handlebars on the tall, skinny racing bike with no brakes and no gears, my life changed forever. I was dressed in an unfamiliar outfit of tight-fitting Lycra, being filmed by *BBC Breakfast* in the Manchester Velodrome on a drab Friday afternoon in winter.

In the autumn of 2012, I had a seemingly innocuous conversation with one of the *Breakfast* producers, Nadia Dahabiyeh. I had no inkling that this short discussion would turn out to be a pivotal moment for me, and would change my life in so many different and exciting ways.

Nadia asked me if I had any ideas for our annual Christmas Challenge. This had become a *BBC Breakfast* tradition: every year in the run-up to Christmas, the presenters were paired up to compete against each other in a variety of challenges. To date they had filmed a version of *Come Dine with Me* at the houses of presenters Susanna Reid and Sian Williams, and a cake baking competition judged by one of the stars of *The Great British Bake* *Off*, Paul Hollywood. The feature was much loved by the *Breakfast* audience and was always hotly contested by the presenters. The Challenge and its results were shown on *Breakfast* in the lead-up to Christmas Day.

December 2012 was going to be the first time I would be involved in the Christmas Challenge. I had become a permanent member of the *Breakfast* presenting team only in April that year, when the programme moved from its base at Television Centre in London to its new home in Salford, MediaCityUK. That year, I would be competing with the other presenters: Bill Turnbull, Susanna Reid and Charlie Stayt.

I had spent much of the summer of 2012, like millions of others, with my eyes glued to the TV watching the London Olympic and Paralympic Games. The haul of gold medals our athletes had won had been inspiring. With that in mind, I suggested to Nadia that perhaps this time, instead of what had been until then cooking challenges, we should plan something to reflect the wonderful summer of sport.

A couple of months later, I had almost forgotten our conversation when she called me to say that she had found the ultimate sporting challenge for us all. We had talked about doing something a bit different, but this was a brilliant, ambitious idea – and much more exciting than I had ever imagined.

She was planning a cycling contest at the home of the hugely successful Great Britain Cycling Team: the Velodrome at the HSBC UK National Cycling Centre in Manchester. The scale of the challenge was epic; none of us had ever cycled in a velodrome before. We would have an Olympic cycling gold medallist to coach us and, if that were not intimidating enough, we would compete in front of a crowd of 4,000 people.

The idea was inspired but terrifying.

The actual race itself was going to be a type of sprint relay, and the rules were very simple. There would be two teams, with two presenters in each team. Each individual rider would race one lap of the 250m track. The finishing times of the riders would be added together, and the team with the faster time would win the *Breakfast* gold medal.

We didn't have a choice about which team we were on – and, to make it even more competitive, the teams were chosen according to our on-screen partnership. So Bill and Susanna, who presented at the start of the working week, would make up one team, and Charlie and I would race together in the other.

The scene was set. A couple of weeks later, just before Christmas, I found myself dressed in what seemed to me ridiculously figure-hugging, bright yellow Lycra. Alongside me were Charlie, Bill and Susanna in the venue where so many of our medal-winning cyclists had trained and raced.

I had never stepped into a velodrome before, nor had I sat on, let alone ridden, a racing bike. My only experience of a velodrome had been watching the Olympics, and shouting at the television as Chris Hoy, Victoria Pendleton, Jason Kenny, Laura Trott, Sarah Storey and their teammates won gold after gold for Team GB in 2012. I found it an exhilarating sport to watch: they all made it look so elegant and easy as they flew round the track, heads down, legs pumping, smashing world records.

I wondered how I would cope. I was nervous, but determined to give it my best shot – and just hoped I wouldn't make a fool of myself or hurt myself by crashing my bike.

The *Breakfast* cycling challenge wasn't going to be a record beater by any means, but it was going to be fun. Before we were allowed on the track, though, and for obvious health and safety reasons, we had to turn up early on a Friday morning for an hour-long training session.

I gasped as I walked into the Velodrome for the first time and caught a glimpse of the intimidating, precipitous bank of wooden boards surrounded by thousands of seats stacked high above them. It was petrifying.

Until then, I had no idea how steep the oval track would be. On television, it had seemed almost flat as I watched cyclists racing at breakneck speeds around it, but it wasn't flat at all – far from it. The gradient of 42° at each end made it look like an alarmingly steep slide, and I was supposed to cycle on a skinny little bike around it. How did anyone stay upright on it, without their bike shooting out from underneath them, let alone reach speeds of 80 km per hour?

My heart beat fast in my chest. I felt claustrophobic and out of breath before I even got to the safety of the apron – or infield, as it's called – in the centre of the track. This is where we were met by our coaches and were presented with a line of bikes racked beside each other, waiting for us to try them.

To calm myself down, one of the first things I did on reaching the side of the track was to see if I could slide down it, on my bottom. Sure enough, as I had imagined, the polished Siberian pine surface and pitched banks meant I whizzed down at high speed, and landed in a heap on the ground, laughing slightly hysterically. Knowing exactly how steep it was, was no comfort at all.

As I picked myself up from the floor, I wondered whether our Olympic gold medallists had ever been so childish and tried out that technique themselves.

The only thing that reassured me was that all four of us were feeling equally afraid now, including the normally supremely confident Charlie Stayt:

'I felt really shaky. I was very nervous of the place, I was daunted by it and the challenge. I was astonished by how steep the slope of the Velodrome was. In my mind's eye, I thought I will be doing that thing where I would be going up the side and swooping down. That's how I thought it was going to be. But when I got there, all I wanted to do was hug the bit where the line is.'

Susanna, who hadn't been on a bike since she was a child, was feeling sick with fear: 'I was absolutely petrified.'

Bill, who still remembers the day clearly, five years on, was also nervous – but more perturbed at being made to wear a pink Lycra top by Susanna (she described him as looking like a baboon in a nappy):

'It seemed to be an exercise in ritual humiliation. My main aim of the day was to make sure that Louise did not beat me. It was a contest that I didn't want to lose, because if I did, I knew a big fuss was going to be made about it, because it was on telly. If I lost, it was going to be even more embarrassing.'

What struck me was how deeply shaken we all were at being removed far from our comfort zone. We could all cope calmly and competently with anything going wrong while we sat on the familiar *BBC Breakfast* red sofa, presenting live in front of more than six million people. But by contrast, in the unfamiliar surroundings of the Velodrome, our cool-headed assurance deserted us. We were all jittery, anxious and scared.

As a bunch of complete amateurs, we found our pre-race coaching session alarming. I seemed to have an overwhelmingly long list of things to understand and then remember.

My first concern was the bike itself.

We were going to be racing on Dolan Track Bikes, which have a fixed gear ratio. This meant they have no free wheel, and you can't coast. If the bike is moving, the pedals are turning – whether you want them to or not.

That was bad enough, but it was made more frightening by knowing that we were going to be wearing cycling shoes, which clipped onto the pedals. I had seen these but never tried them. The combination of the fixed gear and the clipped-in shoes meant that the only time I could physically stop pedalling was when I was at a complete standstill. To my cost – and agony – I very quickly discovered that if I stopped moving my legs, my feet were dragged round by the pedals, out of my control, as if they didn't belong to me.

Added to that, there were no brakes. No brakes? How was I meant to stop?

I was also really concerned about the saddle and its position. It seemed to be set way too high, making me feel as if I were perched on a precarious narrow parapet, towering above the track. It was absurdly narrow: I could hardly sit on it, let alone balance on it.

I had so many things to think about, I thought I would never make it round the first lap. Eventually, after working out how to attach my shoes on to the pedals and with my cycling helmet securely tightened, I set off, wobbling from side to side.

As I gathered speed, white knuckles holding tight on to the handlebars, I screamed in terror for most of the way around my first loop.

It took me another couple of circuits of the track to work out how to steer properly and – most importantly – how to stop. This seemed to be achieved by slowing down my pedalling and then, at the last moment and just before I toppled over, grabbing a handrail. Slowly, I began to get a little more confident and realised that the faster I went, the safer I felt. The bike seemed to get more grip and traction on the wooden track. By lap three, something had changed: I was beginning to enjoy it. A smile spread across my face and I started going faster.

Susanna was finding it incredibly difficult, describing it as the hardest thing she had ever done and saying she felt like a child learning to ride a bike all over again. She spent a tearful 45 minutes with our coach gently trying to persuade her just to let go of the side rail and put both hands on the handlebars: 'I was clinging to the rails for dear life, talking to the coach as if he was my dad, saying: "Please don't let me fall, I can't let go."'

With only a couple of minutes remaining before our allotted hour was up, she launched herself off gingerly on to the track, and managed to navigate a single lap.

In the meantime, Bill was chasing after me, trying to catch me up. He was puffing so hard from the exertion, he had to be pulled off the track by our coach, who was concerned about how hard he was breathing. Bill was loving it, but admitted later that he had tried a little bit too hard, exhausting himself on the way round.

When we finished our training session, Charlie, who had been nervous at the start, was easily the most confident out of the four of us, and by far the most determined. 'I wanted to win massively. I wanted to beat you, Bill and Susanna. There was no way I was leaving that track not winning. I wanted to leave that place as the fastest on that day.'

Our stressful practice session complete, we had only one day before going back for the Christmas Challenge, and there was nothing I could do in preparation, except to try and get a little bit of sleep. Both Charlie and I would be presenting *Breakfast* on the morning of the race. It's a four-hour programme on a Saturday, preceded by a 3.30 a.m. alarm call, so I knew it was going to be a very long and exhausting day.

Given that it was December, my husband, David, and children, Mia and Scarlett, were going to London for some Christmas shopping and couldn't come with me, but they wished me luck the night before. I tried to give them a sense of the immensity of the adventure, and how nervous I was, but they were completely unfazed, gave me a hug and sent me on my way.

The Velodrome was packed, hot and noisy, and there were cyclists already thundering in packs around the track when we returned for race night. The crowds now filling the stands were enthusiastic and devoted cycling fans. They were there to watch the Revolution Series, a track cycling competition that is the equivalent of a Premiership football match. We were just the warm-up act.

The atmosphere felt oppressive and airless. Wrapped up in skin-tight Lycra, I was breathless, my heart racing before I even stepped down on to the track.

I felt out of place and intimidated. Apart from us amateurs on the *Breakfast* team, all the cyclists seemed to know exactly what they were doing – and I didn't have a clue. They looked so young, fit and focused, and so perfectly in tune with each other, I didn't even dare to speak to any of them, for fear of looking even more like a fool.

Ahead of the race, we had one last chance to ride round the circuit, and check if we could remember anything of what we had learned during training. This time, Ed Clancy, a team pursuit Olympic gold medallist, was there to oversee us. After watching us closely, he lined us up for some last-minute advice.

'Get up to your top speed as quick as you can, and really try and pedal through your legs and your hips, rather than pulling on your bars, because when you do that, your line will all start to go to pot, and you will start losing seconds here or there. Try and keep your elbows in, and try and keep your head down because aerodynamics will start coming into it as well.'

We all listened to him carefully but quizzically, and when he mentioned aerodynamics, I burst into nervous laughter. At our slow speeds, did he really think aerodynamics would make any difference? And how were we going to remember any of what he had said? Seeing how incredulous we were, he changed his words to a much simpler version, one that we could all remember: 'Just pedal really hard.'

Perfect, just the kind of instruction I was capable of following.

With half an hour to go before the race, Bill was talking a big game, determined that he wouldn't be beaten by me. Much to his frustration and annoyance, I had been slightly faster than him in practice. Playing up for our *BBC Breakfast* camera, he declared, 'There is one promise I have made myself, I can't be beaten by a girl.'

Susanna was still very nervous and trembling visibly. 'I was convinced I was going to come flying off the bike and it would land on top of me. I was so worried that, although everyone else was just kitted out in their Lycra, I wore long sleeves and leggings underneath mine, as I was trying to protect my arms and legs when I fell.'

Charlie was ashen-faced and admitted that his legs had turned into jelly, and I felt like I had a swarm of butterflies doing somersaults in my stomach.

At that point, it was clear there was a lot of pride at stake here. We each had our own individual goals, and they didn't coincide. Charlie wanted to beat all of us; Bill wanted to beat me; I wanted to beat Bill; and Susanna wanted to get home without crashing and hurting herself.

I knew that Charlie's lap time was going to be very important to me, as our combined times would decide whether it was us or Susanna and Bill who would clinch the title.

With the commentary from cycling legend Hugh Porter echoing around the Velodrome, and Ed Clancy as our outrider, the race began.

Bill went first, cheered on loudly by the raucous crowd.

He had a look of steely determination. There was a slight wobble at the start, but he gritted his teeth, put his head down and pushed as hard as he could. He even had the presence of mind to dip for the line. He whizzed round in 23.832 seconds, and then did a victory lap, waving one hand high in the air.

He had looked fantastic and fast, and I was worried. I also couldn't believe we were being timed to hundredths of seconds. Was that necessary? But in track cycling, fractions of a second count. When it comes to it, milliseconds can make the difference between a winner and a loser.

Charlie was next to start. Resolutely determined to win, he set off at a blistering pace. Extremely focused, with his head swaying, mouth wide open and gasping for air, he accelerated, driving his legs as hard as he possibly could.

'I was furiously intent to the point of reckless disregard for my own health. Genuinely, as I was nearing the end, I thought: This is the closest I have come to a cardiac arrest in my entire lifetime. I thought: This could be it!'

His heroic effort paid off, and he stormed round the track in a very impressive 20.515 seconds. A stunning three seconds faster than Bill.

Halfway through the race, we, the Yellow Team, were well ahead of our opponents.

The question was, could Susanna conquer her fear, get herself round the track, and scrape back some time for Bill?

Despite the paralysing nerves she had suffered in practice, she pulled herself together. Taking a deep breath, she set off steadily and gracefully, her ponytail waving behind her. She managed to look both glamorous and serene, but though she appeared outwardly calm, she was feeling the pressure.

'I felt it was a bit like *Strictly Come Dancing*, it was incredibly intense. With 4,000 people watching, you have a choice: you can bottle it and not do it, or you rise to the occasion, go for it, and throw yourself into it. The crowd were so supportive, cheering us all the way around. I felt like I was surfing on the energy of the crowd, and it wrapped me in a happy cloud.'

Despite her fears and earlier tears, and buoyed by the crowd, Susanna sailed round the track in a respectable 26 seconds. But successfully crossing the finish line didn't mean she was safe.

'I was so grateful to have made it round, not to have fallen off and suffered a catastrophic injury, that when I was slowing down, I lost the plot at the end, and lost control of the bike, and veered straight up the side. I had that sick feeling with a rush of adrenaline, and just managed to force the bike back under control.'

Luckily for me, I didn't see Susanna's perilous helter-skelter finish. I was already poised, one hand on the safety rail and ready to let go. I know if I had seen her nearly fall, it would have filled me with terror and I would have lost my nerve.

As things stood, unless I completely messed it up, Charlie and I would most likely be taking home the *BBC Breakfast* Christmas Challenge title. That mattered, but what mattered most to me right then was to race fast enough to beat Bill – and make sure he was, as he had been fearing all day, 'beaten by a girl'.

I took a last deep breath, closed my eyes for a half-second to focus, and when I was given the signal to go, gripped tightly on the handlebars, drove my legs with all my might, and headed straight towards the red sprinters' line, shadowed by Ed Clancy like a hawk, flying on his bike right beside me.

In that second I let go of the rail, the butterflies were gone. In their place was a steely resolve to knuckle down, go for it, and try as hard as I could.

I pushed the pedals using every ounce of strength, gasping for breath. All I could see was the track unfolding in front of me; all I could hear, my pulse beating loudly in my ears. The crowd roared, my legs burned and my heart raced.

Instead of screaming like I did during the practice, I had a huge wide grin on my face. I was nearly sick with the effort, but I loved it.

I loved it.

The exhilaration as I flashed past the finish line was overwhelming. With momentum carrying me on, I cycled another lap, overexcited and waving giddily to the spectators. I felt a shot of pure adrenaline: I loved the race, I loved going fast, and I wanted to do it all over again.

But had I beaten Bill?

My time flashed up on the scoreboard.

23.378 seconds.

To my surprise and utter delight, I had done it. I had crossed the line just under half a second ahead of Bill. Brilliant! The most exhilarating, satisfying and memorable half-second of my life.

Unsurprisingly, watching my time flash up on the giant screen above him, Bill was gutted, and couldn't cover up his disappointment for the cameras.

'She beat me? Surely not? No! *No!* Ah, that hurts!'

I was on such a high that our medal ceremony was a bit of a blur. We were hustled on to the podium in the centre of the track, all still hobbling because we were wearing our cycling shoes. Lizzie Deignan, road race Olympic silver medallist, was there to award us our medals as the wonderful crowd gave us a cheer.

I was ecstatic. I had never won a 'gold medal' before – it didn't matter that it was a home-made *BBC Breakfast* one. I felt like I had triumphed at the Olympic Games, and I wanted to do it all over again. It was as if a spark went off in my brain and changed me there and then. I had been forced to step out of my comfort zone – and unexpectedly, out of the blue, had come face to face with something incredible.

When I look back now, and watch the moment I let go of the rail to start the race, it is an extraordinary sensation. It's like watching a critical junction in my life, where I made a decision that changed me for ever. I had no idea at the time; it is only with hindsight that I can see how important the moment was, and how profoundly it affected me.

It could have been completely different.

Charlie and I already had his astonishing time in the bag. In the moment I let go of my grasp on the safety rail, I could have made the decision to take it easy, get around the track safely and still have gone home with that gold medal. But that is not the choice I made. In that split second, something switched in my brain, and my competitive spirit, which had been latent for nearly 30 years, was reignited.

I put my heart on the line. This was the moment I was going to go for it, do my best, try my hardest and give it, yes, 100 per cent.

Susanna could see the effect it had on me much more clearly at the time.

'You took to it like a duck to water. You sat on that bike and it was like you fitted together. You immediately sat a little taller, and I could see you grow in confidence, you came alive in that moment. It was like an epiphany for you. You had found your thing, and it was obvious that you weren't just going to do this only as a fun *BBC Breakfast* challenge. This was something you knew you could do and you would do again. It was magic and inspiring to see it and be part of it.'

That night, after winning the gold medal, I left the Velodrome a completely different person.

The pure joy, excitement and rush of endorphins shook me up. It forced me to remember how much I loved sport, how much I loved to race, and to realise that I should never have given it up decades earlier.

That was it, I was hooked. Aged 44, and nearly 30 years after my last swimming competition, I wanted to start all over again and immerse myself in competitive sport.

What exactly I would do, I had no idea. I just knew that I had to do something.

CHAPTER 2

SOME OF THE GEAR, NO IDEA

'You run and you cycle. Have you ever thought about doing a triathlon?'

Katie Moore, neighbour

We left the Velodrome in the dark. On the way home, I was euphoric with adrenaline and excitement, calling my family and talking nineteen to the dozen about every single detail. I had loved the whole thing: the jangling nerves before the race; the intense, almost suffocating atmosphere; my heart racing before the starting bell; the roar of the crowd; those moments of extreme effort pumping my legs as hard as I could, lungs bursting; the exhilaration of speed, wind and shouts thundering in my ears; and the pure delight as I flew over the finish line. I was over the moon to have beaten Bill, but it wasn't that which I loved the most, it was the race itself.

The post-race buzz lasted for days, and it didn't leave when we played the race report over two days on *Breakfast*. Normally I cringe when I watch myself back on TV, but scrutinising the unfolding story, it was obvious that something had changed in me. The joy and excitement on my face was plain for everyone to see.

When I eventually came down from the Velo-high, the first thing I resolved to do was to start looking for a bike. My old faithful bike, which I had treasured on the commute from Wandsworth to work at Television Centre in west London, had been stolen when we moved to Chester. I would have to start again from scratch. But a road bike with a measly six gears, or even a mountain bike, wasn't what I wanted to ride any more; I wanted a bicycle for racing. Quite where I was going to race, I had no idea, but that wasn't going to stop me.

My family thought I was mad. I had only ever ridden a bike for the commute into work, presenting on the BBC News Channel. That was six or so miles, and more often than not, to make it easier, I would hop on the train with the bike on the way there or the way back, so I very seldom actually rode the 12-mile round trip. As a result, they were perplexed when I said I wanted a bike to start racing – and sceptical that I would ever actually ride it, let alone race it.

My first stop was at a local bike shop. They were brilliant at dealing with a total novice, asking me in detail what I wanted the bike for, explaining how the gears worked, and showing me how to clip cycling shoes into the metal pedals.

Luckily the shop had a huge car park, so I tried out different road bikes, dodging around parked cars. Sitting high above the handlebars on a tiny seat felt very precarious, and the slightest movement of my hands made it turn alarmingly sharply. The gears and brakes seemed to be scarily out of easy reach, and the tyres dangerously narrow. Nevertheless, I left with a white Kona Zing Supreme with flashy orange and black stripes, plus a ridiculous amount of new kit – all carefully placed in the back of the car. Padded Lycra cycling shorts, a cycle top with pockets on the back, bike gloves, and a new snazzy white cycle helmet to match my bike – I spent a small fortune. David, my husband, was horrified and kept saying: Are you sure you're going to use it? But nothing would stop me; I couldn't wait.

The first few tentative bike rides on my new set of very skinny wheels were nervy experiences. I wobbled dangerously across the road as I tried to fix my bike shoes into the cleats, looking down to see if I was at least aiming my foot in the right direction. Apart from the Velodrome, I had never used drop handlebars. They seemed needlessly far away from me, and very low. I was only happy with my hands on the top of the handlebars, not on the drop handlebars. Either way, trying to reach the brakes and change gear was extremely challenging.

Also – and I know this sounds completely ridiculous – I had no idea how to get off the bike properly. I was so paranoid about having my shoes stuck in the cleats and then toppling over, unable to get my foot down to the safety of the ground, that I would take both feet out several metres away from any junction and then balance precariously on the seat until I slowed down enough to lean over and rest a foot on the floor. Not at all ladylike, really quite painful and, to anyone who happened to see me, the sure sign that I was a total amateur.

What you are meant to do – and I found this out only years later and after several grazed knees – is to take one foot out, lean forward with the other leg bent so that your free foot is closer to the ground, glide to a graceful gentle safe stop, place your free foot down gently, and then unclip and take the other foot out! So simple when you know how.

Slowly, after several excursions, the wobbles began to ease and I started to gather a little bit of speed – just what I had been after ever since my Velodrome adventure. In London, though, I had ridden my bike round the city very slowly, and was so unaccustomed to going at any sort of pace that at first I thought the wind buzzing in my ears was the sound of an engine. Every time I gathered any momentum, I kept imagining there were cars right behind me, and would glance over my shoulder to check that I wasn't in the way.

My confidence grew slowly with small forays into the wonderful but challenging Welsh hills and I realised my Velodrome revelation was spot on: I loved cycling for cycling's sake. Loved being outside, wind in my ears, wheels rolling and whizzing my way through the countryside. For the first time in years, I was just 'doing', and enjoying the 'doing', and not thinking and worrying about a thing. All I was thinking about, if I was even thinking at all, was the noise of the wheels, the angle of the sunlight, the smoothness of the road, and where I might stop to have a cup of tea and eat a piece of cake – something I quickly learned was an essential part of cycling.

I was enjoying it so much that after a couple of months I managed to persuade David to buy a bike too. When we could, while the children were at school and we had both finished work, we spent happy hours cycling together, mostly in search of nice pubs to stop for a quick pint for him and lunch for me.

Things stepped up a gear – literally – when I bumped into Katie Moore, a friend who lives in the same village. Not only had she watched the Christmas Challenge, she had also seen me out on my bike and running along the banks of the River Dee with my golden Labrador, Waffle. 'You run and you cycle,' she said. 'Have you ever thought about doing a triathlon? I've signed up for one in Chester, why don't you do it with me?'

The embarrassing thing is, I didn't really have much of a clue at the time what a triathlon was. I thought it involved cycling, swimming and running, and I knew that the Brownlees, a couple of brothers from Yorkshire, were really good at it and had won medals in the Olympics. Beyond that, it was a fog: I was less than sure about the order for doing the different activities, and certainly had no idea of how you went from one to the other or how far you had to race. That didn't deter me. If Katie was going to give it a go, so was I. I knew I could swim (I had been reasonably good at school); I was loving the cycling; and although I didn't much like running, I could do so if necessary. So, I signed up with four or five months to go and then set about trying to train.

The race Katie had chosen was the Deva Divas, an award-winning and much loved women's-only race set on the Meadows below the historic city of Chester. It has the convenient bonus of being only a couple of miles from where I live. The race begins with a 750-metre swim downstream in the River Dee. This is followed by a 25-kilometre bike ride from the Meadows, out of the ancient city, along to the border with Wales and back again. It then finishes with a 5-kilometre run beside the Dee.

Part of the ethos behind the race is to help encourage women into the sport who have never done a triathlon before. It is designed to be accessible to all levels of experience, and all shapes and sizes. Whether you have never been swimming in open water, or ride an ancient bike with a shopping basket attached to the front, or fancy yourself as an up-and-coming triathlete, the Deva Divas is perfect for you. Thankfully, the Chester Triathlon Club also organised a series of Deva Divas training days, for novice triathletes like me. The women who arrived for the training day presented a huge range of ages and abilities. Some of them were a bit wobbly on their bikes and looked like they had done even less cycling than I had, but others looked like accomplished athletes and speedy runners.

Even turning up for a training session was daunting. We met by the river with our bikes in various states of chaos, and then set off in small groups to try out the cycle route. Just getting on the bike was a challenge; the start was up a steep hill, which meant it was virtually impossible to get your feet clipped into the pedals. To save embarrassment, I pushed it up the hill the first time rather than fall over and make a fool of myself.

Coaches from Chester Triathlon Club escorted us along the way, cycling along beside us, giving us gentle hints about our riding technique, and telling us what sort of thing to look out for. They told us to watch out for holes and bumps in the road, and how to take a hand off the handlebars so that we could point at the problem to help riders behind us.

I loved my first ride out on the route, and was feeling pretty chuffed with myself for having managed to keep up with the group. So chuffed that I sped down the hill at the end, came to a successful sharp stop in front of about twenty other wannabe triathletes, gave them a huge smile and said: 'Wasn't that great?' – then toppled over on my side!

I had forgotten to take my feet out of the cleats – the rookie mistake. There I was, stuck like an upside-down tortoise and still attached to the bike. I grazed my elbow and knee, but it was my pride that suffered the most damage. I laughed, and hoped the others would think it was funny, but they looked at me in pity, and watched as I tried to wriggle out from under my bike pretending it hadn't hurt.

The triathlon club also took us on a swimming excursion that day. I love swimming, and I particularly love swimming outdoors in lakes or in the sea, but this time I was lowering myself into the muddy brown water of the River Dee. The experience was a heart-stopping one. All of us triathlon newbies gingerly climbed down the water's edge, gripped each other's hands for support as we stepped carefully over some barbed wire, and then launched ourselves into the cold dark water. This was not a swim for the faint-hearted to attempt.

I was properly prepared for the water, having bought myself a triathlon wetsuit. These might look similar to surf wetsuits but are more stretchy and flexible so they don't restrict your arm movements when you are swimming. They also tend to have more neoprene on the legs to help with buoyancy in the water, and have an especially long and accessible zip so that you can reach it easily, pull it down fast, and take it off quickly when you have finished the swim and are ready to mount your bike.

The Tri Club were taking no risks with their fledgling triathletes, and had kayaks out on the river to assist us. That didn't stop my breath being taken away by the shock of getting in, far out of my depth and knowing that there were metres of deep black water flowing fast beneath me. Quite rightly, the Tri Club insists on swimming with a wetsuit, and I have never been more glad of one – not so much for the warmth but for the feeling that it was helping me keep afloat. My first afternoon in the river, we swam only 400 metres – and that was quite enough for me. On the day of the Triathlon, the distance would be nearly double.

The experience of the Deva training day was a bit of a shock to me, and a stark and timely reminder of how clueless I was about triathlon. I had assumed that because I could swim in a pool, I could swim in a river. I had been loving cycling but my fall demonstrated that I was still very much an amateur, and the short jog afterwards confirmed what I already knew – I really didn't like running, and it was much worse after a bike ride.

I could swim, cycle and run, but the thought of putting them all together in a race was extremely daunting. I was so worried that I was going to make an idiot of myself, I asked one of the Chester Tri coaches I had met on the training day, Kelly Crickmore, if she could help. She started by asking me what I wanted to achieve, and I told her my goal was to be able to finish the race, and as a bonus try to enjoy it on the day. With that in mind, Kelly put together a training programme with a couple of runs, bike rides and swims every week for me to complete. It added up to about five hours of training a week.

Looking back now at my training for the 5-kilometre run, I find it hard to understand why it seemed so difficult at the time; I can only compare it to how far I can run now. And yet five kilometres seemed a very long way.

This probably reflected my earlier experience. In 2005, when my daughter Mia was about four, I was training for the Great North Run, and she was cycling beside me on her bike with stabilisers. For some reason, I managed to trip over – just missing her. I fell badly, twisting my ankle. I was in agony at the time, but pretended it was OK as I hobbled home, and put on a brave face. It was incredibly bruised and painful, and I just assumed that if I stopped training, it would get better.

It didn't. The aches and pains persisted, which I continued to try and ignore. Eventually, about six years later, when the pain had progressed to my hip and I couldn't sleep because of it, I saw a specialist. To my surprise, an MRI scan revealed that all those years ago, I had done a David Beckham and broken a metatarsal in my right foot. I should have rested and protected it until it had healed, but instead, I had carried on. That meant my whole right side was very weak, and running on my injured foot was still very painful years later.

But I was determined: the small matter of a sore foot wasn't going to stop me attempting my first triathlon. I plodded my way through the runs, and very slowly started being able to run a little bit further, and a tiny bit faster.

CHAPTER 3

NO NUDITY

'You can't win a race in transition, but if you mess it up, you could definitely lose one.'

Apart from the run, cycle and swim training, there was so much to learn about triathlon.

As the weeks ticked down to the race, I realised that it is not a case of successfully competing in three different sports. You also have to change very quickly from one type of exercise to something completely different, in as short a time as possible. So, when you get out of the water sopping wet and often freezing cold, you must rip off your wetsuit, hat and goggles, stuff your ice-cold feet into cycle shoes, push your bike to the mount line, jump on it, and get a move on! If you want to race competitively, there is no time to hang about to dry yourself with a towel, or to bother putting on your socks. Elite triathletes like Alistair and Jonathan Brownlee take it a step further than I have ever dared, and have their cycle shoes already clipped on to their pedals. They manage to jump on the bike and fasten their feet in while already on the move.

That short changeover is called 'transition' in the Triathlon world, and there are all sorts of rules that you must obey. For example, you can be disqualified if you touch your bike before you have your helmet on and the strap done up – a rule that is very sensible from a safety perspective. Other errors can result in being given a time penalty to serve out later in the race – discarding your soggy wetsuit on the ground, for example, rather than in the plastic box that is sometimes provided.

One of my absolute favourite rules, which seems to apply to lots of races, is 'no nudity'. Every time I read it in the rules, it makes me laugh out loud; I can't imagine why anyone would want to get naked in the middle of what is normally a field surrounded by lots of spectators.

The tight rules can cause all sorts of problems. Even the most experienced triathletes and top-level competitors have been known to make mistakes.

Jonathan Brownlee, now an Olympic silver medallist, was given a 15-second penalty at London 2012 for mounting his bike just a fraction of a second too early. Despite that, he still managed to hold on to the bronze medal in the race. Non Stanford, one of Team GB's top triathletes and World Champion in 2013, has twice been given penalties for not putting her wetsuit in the correct box in transition.

Such strict rules are one of the reasons I love the sport. You can train all you like, but on race-day anything can happen; there is so much that can go wrong. My theory goes: You can't win a race in transition, but if you mess it up, you could definitely lose one!

Thankfully, the Deva coaches had transition covered, and on those training days talked us through exactly how to approach it.

Be incredibly organised: before you even get to the race start, you should have all your kit together for the three different events. Wetsuit, swimming goggles, sunglasses, water bottles, cycle shoes, running shoes, etc. You must also check, of course, that your bike is race-ready, tyres pumped and brakes working.

Once you have arrived at the race, registered and made your way to transition, you must work out where to put everything. The ideal set-up would make it as easy as possible for you to find the right thing at the right time. You don't want to be scrabbling for your helmet or your lucky sunglasses under a pile of shoes.

In transition, each athlete has a small space, normally under or right beside their bike, to lay out their equipment. For me, what's most important is to make sure I make it impossible to get myself disqualified. I always put my bike helmet on my handlebars, so I can't possibly fail to see it and put it on before I touch the bike. I also put my sunglasses in the helmet, again so that I can't fail to see them and put them on.

Ahead of that first race, the Deva Divas coaches made us practise transition. I did a few dummy runs at home, laying out all my things in the right place and rehearsing the change from swim to bike to run.

Five months after that initial conversation with Katie, and with hours of swimming, running and cycling under my belt, as well as all the different rules now straight in my head, I was just about ready to give it a go.

CHAPTER 4

MY FIRST TRIATHLON

'I could tell by the expression on David's face that he was worried about me, and he was absolutely right to be. I was in trouble.'

I was fit. But I wasn't ready for the race.

Having not done any competitive sport since I gave up swimming at the age of 15, nearly 30 years before, I had completely forgotten that I have a love-hate relationship with race-day.

It always starts with hate. First, I have great difficulty sleeping and then I wake up with butterflies flying round my stomach. I can hardly even look at food, let alone eat. I keep losing things. I am fidgety. I talk utter nonsense. In fact, I am extremely annoying.

The day of my first race, I got myself into such a fluster that, despite living only 10 minutes away from the start line, I arrived late at the registration tent. By the time I had packed everything into the car and gone back at least twice for the things I thought I had forgotten (and hadn't), I was way behind.

When I finally made it to the grassy patchwork of wetlands known as the Meadows beside the River Dee, I breathlessly pushed my bike to the small section of field cordoned off for transition. I made it with only seconds to spare before it was closed for the race to begin. There was an impressive turnout: more than 250 female competitors and double the amount of spectators milling about, with triathlon kit strewn all over the place. Realising the chaotic state I was in, a marshal took pity on me and helped me find my spot, racking my bike on the metal A-frame above me while I pulled things randomly out of my bag, shoving them underneath the bike in no semblance of order. So much for race planning, and having a chance to check it all over! That's what the pressure of an event can do.

Katie was there an hour before me, and was very organised, with her wetsuit on and ready to go. She seemed to be an oasis of calm compared to the bundle of nerves that I was. We had a last photo taken together before we began the long and nervy walk upstream to the start. In the chaos, I had forgotten to pack any flip-flops or other shoes except my running shoes, which were now stored in transition, so I had to pick my way carefully over the gravel in bare feet.

The one thing I had been feeling quietly confident about was the swim. Every time I trained in the pool, I swam more than 2,000 metres easily, so I thought that a mere 750 metres, with the current carrying me downstream, should be a doddle. I tried to listen to the safety briefing, but the nerves made it difficult to concentrate. The only thing I remembered hearing was: If you are in trouble, lie on your back, wave, and someone will come to help.

One by one, we gingerly stepped down the bank into the river towards the start. This was an imaginary line between two huge buoys about 10 metres apart in the river, beneath the pretty houses and immaculate gardens tumbling down the hill to the riverbank on this unseasonably chilly July day.

The water felt icy as I put my feet, knees and hands into it, and I shivered as it slowly filled up my wetsuit, inch by inch, taking my breath away. Unlike my first swim in the Dee, it was shallow enough to stand, and I watched with my arms folded around me to keep out the cold, as the serious triathletes got straight in: no messing about, they started a warm-up front crawl. I wasn't going to do any of that. They were graceful and fast, and they looked like they were being driven along by invisible propellers underneath the water; swimming was no effort at all. Doubts flooded into my head: maybe I wasn't as good at swimming as I had thought, maybe the whole race was a bad idea.

I looked back to the shore, to give one more forced smile to my husband, David. He was waiting and waving with my two daughters, Mia and Scarlett, who were dressed in warm coats and sheltering under the trees. Waffle, our one-year-old golden Labrador puppy, was straining on her lead, wagging her tail enthusiastically and trying to work out where I had disappeared to.

With the last few seconds to go, we jostled for places. Then all of a sudden we were off, in a blinding flurry of kicking feet and flailing arms. There seemed to be wetsuited women everywhere – in front of me, behind me, beside me, on top of me. I couldn't get my breath, couldn't see anything; felt claustrophobic and scared. Desperate for air, I floundered my way out of the mêlée into clearer water and tried to get my stroke into some sort of rhythm, but l couldn't get my breath back. For the first time in my life I was panicking in the water, and it was terrifying.

For some semblance of security, I concentrated on hugging the riverbank, keeping myself alongside, parallel with it, as I struggled to keep on swimming. After what seemed like a lifetime gulping for air, and feeling as if I couldn't remember how to swim, I caught a glimpse of a yellow streak that was Waffle, and realised I could see familiar feet rushing along beside me. It was David and the girls jogging along the riverbank. I could tell by the expression on David's face that he was worried about me, and he was absolutely right to be. I was in trouble.

Between my snatched breaths, I managed to shout to him, 'How far to go?'

'You're halfway there!' was the shout back. Only halfway! That wasn't what I expected. I felt like I had already swum 2,000 metres, not just 350.

Between gasps, I fixed my eyes on the kicking feet of another swimmer a few metres in front of me. Focused on her, I kept up as best I could, occasionally checking where the safety buoys were, and if she was guiding me in the right direction.

Eventually, after what seemed long minutes of pure panic, my breathing calmed down a bit. Then, to my relief and after what seemed an eternity, I saw a flash of white: Chester's Iron Bridge ahead of me. I knew the finish was somewhere between where I was and the bridge, so I was nearly there. I gave a final push, and was ecstatic to successfully navigate my way to the jetty, where I was hauled to my feet by a couple of wonderful volunteers, spluttering, dizzy and wobbling.

My feet were frozen, but my head was clear. As soon as I was out of the water, I felt a million times better. I began to focus on the race itself, rather than being in a blind panic. All the training and practice started paying off as I remembered how to take off my wetsuit, hauling down the zip and dragging it down. I took care not to touch my bike, or take it off the rack before I had my helmet on and safely fastened.

Compared to the swim, the cycle ride was a joy. I loved every second of it. I didn't care that my tri suit, which I had been wearing like a seasoned triathlete under my wetsuit, was soaking wet. I just loved being out on the road and cycling like a lunatic. The support on the course was fantastic, with people shouting and waving at us as we whizzed through villages and past houses. The 25 kilometres flashed past and I even managed to catch up, then overtook a couple of fellow Deva competitors on the way. I scooted into transition a mere 52 minutes later with a huge grin on my face. The ride had been brilliant fun.

I tried as quickly as I could to rack my bike, so I could change into my running shoes and get out of transition. Disaster! Try as I might, I couldn't work out how I was meant to balance my bike on the metal bar. Every time I did it – and I tried about five times – it just fell off. I felt like such a fool. Because I had been so late into transition and the marshal had racked my bike for me, I had no idea that you simply hook the front of the seat over the metal bar and there it stays. Incredibly easy if you know how to do it. As I was faffing about, another triathlete rushed in to rack her bike, and I watched as she neatly put the seat into the right place and ran out in front of me.

Now came the run. I had imagined that after the bike ride it might be hard. Even so, I was completely unprepared for my legs turning into concrete blocks that were out of my control. I had been warned to practise running after getting off my bike, but I had never quite found the time. My reasoning had been that I didn't like running anyway, so how or why would the triathlon run be any worse than normal?

It was much worse!

There are lots of theories about why the bike–run transition is so hard. Some people say it's because you use different muscle groups cycling compared to running and these take a while to adapt. Or it could simply be fatigue; you are tired after the ride. Right then, I didn't care why it was happening, just that it was happening, and that I was in agony.

The only upside was that being back on the Meadows meant my family could run beside me – a huge bonus. They were brilliant!

Scarlett, who was then only eight years old, ran along next to me, shouting wonderful words of encouragement: 'Come on, Mummy, you can do this.'

I felt like a wounded giraffe as I hobbled on hopeless, heavy legs round the course. I tried to force myself to go faster, but the second loop was almost too much for me. When Mia and Scarlett couldn't see me at the far end, I slowed right the way down to a walk, with a screeching painful stitch right across my right shoulder and chest paralysing one side.

I wasn't going to give up, though. So an hour and a half after I started, I stumbled across the finish line – gasping for air, falling into the arms of my family, and bursting into floods of tears.

The tears were a surprise to me; I hardly ever cry. What made me so emotional was, I think, a heady mixture of exhaustion, and relief that it was all over, and elation that I had done it. I was shattered, but after a large piece of home-made cake given to me by the race volunteers and more hugs from my family, I very quickly started feeling better.

That afternoon, for the first time in my fledgling sporting career, I was handed a tiny slip of paper with my results. In my very first triathlon, I had come 43rd out of 273 competitors. Even though the swim had felt like a frightening struggle, I had swam the 750 metres in a respectable 14.02 minutes. It turned out that the joy I had felt while cycling had been mirrored in my speed: I had finished the 25 kilometres in 52.32 minutes. Then, and even with my post-cycling leaden legs, I had managed the 5-kilometre run in 26.44. An overall time with the transitions of 1.35.12. Not bad for a first-time triathlete.

But most excitingly for me, in my age group I had come eighth. That was the most brilliant revelation to me. Until then, I had no idea that your race times are compared against competitors who are the same age as you. So, unless you are super-fast or an elite triathlete, age is how most triathletes measure their success – where they come in their age group. To me, seventh in the 45–50 age group seemed like a great place to be.

As I gathered up my triathlon kit, strewn about in transition, my thoughts were already turning to the possibility of another race. There were moments when I had been extremely scared, others when I had been nearly overwhelmed and in agony, but the overriding feeling was one of pride and achievement: I had done what I set out to do.

Heading home that day, I already knew I wanted to race again.

CHAPTER 5

KILL OR CURE

'Hurry up, Daddy! Row quickly. Quickly – she's swimming away from us.'

Mia and Scarlett, my daughters

After that first triathlon, I was high on adrenaline for days afterwards, but perplexed about why the river swim had been so scary.

The swimming should have been by far my easiest discipline because I used to compete at school, but this was the moment when I had been most worried. My husband couldn't understand it either. He had seen quite clearly from the bank that I was flailing about, gasping for breath, and not streamlined like I normally am in the pool or the sea.

It took me a few hours, but I soon worked out why I had been so short of breath and panicky. It was because the River Dee is so murky that you can't see your elbow in the water in front of you, let alone your hand. As a result, I felt like I was swimming virtually blind, with no idea of the direction in which I was heading. The lack of visibility had made me feel claustrophobic and nervous, pushing up my heart rate and making me gasp for my breath. Once in a state of panic, I had found it impossible to calm down and get my breath back.

The experience didn't put me off, though. I continued to train, running and cycling but mostly swimming – in the clear blue waters of an indoor pool. Open water, and the fear accompanying it, was not part of the routine.

A few months later, I came across a challenge that might, I thought, be a kill or cure. Walking with Waffle by the river, I saw a tiny poster tied to a wooden post, advertising a long-distance swimming race. The Bridge to Bridge open-water swim was being organised in memory of a local man, Dr Dave Casson. A keen open-water swimmer, he had worked at Alder Hey Children's Hospital and the Countess of Chester Hospital. He had died after a short illness aged 45, and his friends were now organising the race in commemoration as well as to raise money for charity.

There were two choices of distance: 10 kilometres, which is the swimming equivalent of a marathon, or a still daunting 5 kilometres (a half-marathon).

I reckoned that if I attempted to swim five kilometres in the River Dee, the same stretch of water where I had struggled for my first triathlon, then one of two things would happen. Either I would be cured, once and for all, of any worries about open water; or I would never swim in a murky river again. Just running five kilometres in the triathlon had been challenging, but I was deluded enough to think that swimming five kilometres was possible.

I did a few calculations about how long I thought it would take me to swim 5 kilometres in a pool. On a good day, I worked out that it would take somewhere between one and three-quarter hours and two hours. How bad could that be?

I signed up.

What I didn't consider was that this would be nothing like swimming in a warm clear indoor pool, where I could touch the floor and hold on to the side for a breather. The two hours would be in cold, dark, deep water, where I was unable to reach the bottom, and had nothing to hold on to for safety or a rest.

There were a couple of conditions for those taking part in the race, one of which was that all swimmers had to have a supporting boat or kayak alongside, one without a motor. We didn't have a kayak, but we did have a rather unwieldy Avon inflatable, so I reckoned David could row beside me.

To prepare for the race, I did a few long swims in the sea while we were on holiday in North Cornwall. I say long, but the most I ever swam for was about 25 minutes before I got too tired and left the water. David did no rowing training at all.

On the day of the swim, I woke up overexcited and nervous and extremely daunted by the long race ahead. I was ready to go in my wetsuit, and we were just about to launch our boat when we were told about Rule No. 2. I could race only if my support boat was flying a Flag Alpha. Neither of us had a clue what that was, but the swim was being run under British Long Distance Swimming Association rules:

'BLDSA rules require that Flag Alpha is flown by all craft escorting individual swimmers. Flag Alpha is a maritime signal flag that when flown on its own indicates a vessel has a diver down or swimmer in the water. Other craft are expected to give a wide berth and proceed at slow speed. It is recommended that Flag Alpha is mounted on a short pole and attached to the boat. Flag Alpha must be removed if the swimmer retires.'

This had been described in the pre-race notes, but in my haste to take part in the race, I had failed to notice it. When we arrived on the riverbank that morning, the race official made it clear that there was no way I could take part without a Flag Alpha flying on our boat. We asked desperately if one of the organisers or any of the other competitors had a flag that we could borrow – but no one had a spare. Determined not to be defeated before I had even dipped a toe in the water, we made a mad dash home, looked up images of Flag Alpha, cut up a piece of A4 paper, used the children's paint to daub some blue on it in the right shape, and, with the paint still wet, went back and attached it with a bamboo garden stick and some Sellotape to the front of the inflatable. Hey presto! We weren't exactly shipshape, but were ready to go.

Having rushed back to the race event, David and the girls cast themselves out onto the Dee, precariously balancing in the boat. Meanwhile, I stood shivering with about 10 other competitors, mostly women, waiting for the start. (The majority of the men had opted for the 10-kilometre swim.) I had never met any of them before. Only three out of the ten of us were wearing wetsuits; the other brave souls were just sporting their swimming costumes, joking that I might be wearing neoprene but they were wearing 'celluprene', referring proudly to their cellulite. I admired their courage, and thought they were amazingly brave to face the water in just their cossies.

Of all the mad things I have done, the swim has to be one of the most ridiculous. There I was – shivering, barefoot and up to my ankles in mud – and my destination, Chester, was a whopping five kilometres away. The lazy river sliding past us was still the same murky chocolate brown that had scared me before, and the trees thickly lining the steep banks, with branches touching the water, looked like a formidable wall on either side. It would be difficult to scrabble out if I panicked.

At that point in a long race, I find it is always best not to think about the journey ahead, but just to think about the start. I made my way hesitantly into the chilly river, and waited patiently for a couple of minutes, treading water. When the whistle blew, I set off confidently downstream towards Chester, at a fast but steady pace and with the wide river stretching out in front of me. Behind us was a mini flotilla of kayaks, plus our inflatable boat, all cheerfully fluttering their blue and white flags.

The swim started surprisingly well. After the first 500 metres or so, I was feeling absolutely fine. The water was just as murky as it had been on that first triathlon, but it wasn't bothering me. I still found it claustrophobic, but this time I was prepared for it, so I wasn't worried or panicky about not being able to see.

Around me, the other swimmers were settling in beside their paddling kayakers, but I couldn't see David and the girls at all. I kept on swimming, and every now and then stopped to take a look behind me to see where they were, but there was no sign of them.

Where had they gone to, and what on earth was I going to do? I knew that to abide by the rules I should be with a boat. To avoid being disqualified, should I stop and get out, or just keep going in the hope that they would catch me?

Unbeknown to me, David was trapped in a nightmare.

He saw me set off at a cracking pace with the faster swimmers. Even rowing as hard as he could, he couldn't stay with me. He found himself stuck right at the back of the pack, behind the slower swimmers alongside their diligent kayakers, all blocking his path towards me. The only way he could safely navigate around them was by going backwards in order to go forwards.

Frantically rowing as fast as he could, he had to head upstream and take a wide detour to the opposite side of the river in the hope of eventually coming down the inside towards me. He was doing his absolute best as Mia and Scarlett shouted: 'Hurry up, Daddy! Row quickly. Quickly – she's swimming away from us.'

At the 1-kilometre mark, I was still doing fine and had almost given up on them ever catching me. Luckily by then, I had been adopted by another swimmer and their kayaking companion, who was happily paddling along and escorting us both downriver.

When they did eventually catch me up, David – who had been expecting a relaxed fun day out with Mia and Scarlett, just floating gently down the river, being pushed by the current – was red-faced, out of breath and furious. The girls were equally unamused, and their frustration and irritation set me off laughing and spluttering in the water. There was I, swimming in the freezing cold and really enjoying it – and there were they, above the water, wrapped up, warm and dry, but struggling. The more I laughed, the angrier I made them, so I had to giggle with my face down in the water, bubbles breaking the surface, so they couldn't see my mirth.

Even when they had caught up, David's difficulties weren't at an end. A strong headwind kept pushing him in the wrong direction, and he was still having a devil of a struggle to keep up with me.

About halfway to Chester, we did eventually reach some kind of happy equilibrium: I settled into a steady pace, and they stayed right beside me, like guardian angels watching over my every stroke. When I took a breath, I would look up to my left to check if they were still there, and the girls would shout encouragement and smile: 'Come on, Mummy, you can do this.'

It turned out that my biggest enemy on the day wasn't what I had presumed – the lack of visibility or the considerable distance. It was an invisible enemy that sneaked up on me: the cold.

I have suffered from what is called Raynaud's phenomenon since I was a child. If you have Raynaud's, you have oversensitive blood vessels in your extremities. The small blood vessels overreact to cold temperatures and become narrower than usual, significantly restricting blood flow. In my case, it affects my hands and feet. When I was a child, the result was horrendous, burning chilblains on my fingers. These days it can mean that if the temperature is slightly cold, even when I am doing something as harmless as shopping in a supermarket, suddenly one or all of my fingers will turn white and go numb – and likewise my toes. This can even be triggered by something as mundane and as far from endurance sport as you can imagine, like getting a packet of peas out of the freezer.

An hour immersed in the chilly River Dee had taken its toll.

I had felt cold from the start, but now, with about two kilometres still to go, my hands and feet were solid blocks of ice. I had no feeling in them at all. And no feeling meant no control. When I was putting my hand in the water to pull against it, I couldn't even force my fingers together, so it was like trying to swim with heavy blocks of ice attached to my arms. I could still just about kick with my feet, but it was like swimming with heavy boots filled with water. I felt ungainly and cumbersome and uncomfortable. My frozen hands and feet were not my main concern, though: I was more worried by the sensation of numbness creeping up my arms towards my chest. I began to worry that this was more than just my normal Raynaud's, and I began to fear that I was getting dangerously cold and edging close to hypothermia.

David was worried too. But apart from stopping me and dragging me into the boat, there was nothing he could do. Words of encouragement were all he could offer.

Mia and Scarlett were brilliant at keeping my spirits up, waving at me every time I looked up as I painstakingly inched my way down the river.

About a mile before the end in Chester, I hit a long straight stretch of water – and, I think, became delirious. My mind started playing tricks on me. Ahead of me I could see the river turn a bend, but my perspective of it, face down in the water and at river level, created an optical illusion. That bend didn't look far to me, but in reality it was hundreds of metres away. I was trying my best to swim towards it – and it didn't seem to be getting any closer.

I felt like I was having a bad dream, one of those nightmares when you are trying to run away from something and your legs take you nowhere. The minutes passed one after another, painfully, achingly slowly. Hand over hand in the water, getting colder and colder, I couldn't see that I was making any progress.

Eventually, after what seemed like hours, but of course wasn't, I turned the unreachable bend. Looking up, I saw the Iron Bridge glinting like an oasis in the sunlight ahead of me, just as it had done in my first triathlon.

I was going to make it. The finish was in my grasp.

All I had to do was keep on moving and I would get there.

I caught a glimpse of another swimmer beginning to catch me up, but after five kilometres in the water I wasn't going to be beaten to the line. I forced my unwilling hands and feet to go faster, and with sheer effort of will dragged myself under the bridge to the finish line, one hour and 40 minutes after I had started.

Hauled out of the water and on to my ice-block feet, I thought I was fine. I wasn't. As I stood up, my vision went and I couldn't see. Blackness was creeping from the corners of my eyes, enveloping me. I was nauseous, dizzy, and about to faint.

A volunteer saw immediately that I wasn't well, sat me down with my head between my knees and wrapped me in an emergency blanket. I don't know what made me nearly faint – the cold, the exertion, or suddenly standing up – but it gave me a real fright and I was shaking like a leaf. After a hot cup of tea with dollops of sugar, my sight cleared. And I was mightily relieved to have a hot shower before the informal awards ceremony.

It turned out that I had come first in the Ladies 5 Kilometres. However, because I had been wearing a wetsuit, the prize went to a lady who had swum the whole way in nothing but a swimming costume. I met her in the changing rooms, where we were trying to warm up, drying ourselves and wrapping up in layers of extra clothes – which was almost impossible to do with numb hands and feet. Like me, she was shivering uncontrollably, but she had loved it, and seemed to be feeling no worse than I was, despite not wearing a warming wetsuit. Good on her, what an amazing feat! How did she cope with the cold?

I had loved the swim and not once did I worry about not being able to see my hands or what was underneath me. It had been a gruelling but brilliant experience, and it would leave a lasting legacy. Never again would I worry about muddy water, not being able to touch the bottom or not being close to the edge. I had also loved crossing the line first in the women's race. Open-water swimming was now added to the growing list of sports in which I wanted to race.

Legend has it that after you have been swimming in the Dee you must drink a can of Coke to kill any bugs you have swallowed on the way. After the race, we all duly did. But that night I took the legend a little further than I think is intended. I thought it implied that anything fizzy would have the same effect. When David and I went out that evening, to a charity dinner raising money for the Lady Taverners, I was offered champagne and drank quite a lot. Just to kill the bugs, you understand!

In the morning, I felt on top of the world! Neither the party nor the swim had left any ill effects. I turned out to be extremely lucky: out of about 30 swimmers on the day, more than half of them were ill afterwards.

So, in my entirely unprofessional experience, I suggest you try Coke, champagne, beer or whatever your sparkly poison is. Try it and, fingers crossed, you'll beat the bugs too.

CHAPTER 6

PORTALOOS AND TANTRUMS

'Come on, Mummy! For goodness' sake, just get in the water, it's nearly the last wave! You're going to miss it altogether.'

Mia, my daughter

The stench in the tiny, stifling-hot plastic Portaloo was overwhelming, and I was sweating profusely in my tight wetsuit, but I was determined I was not going to come out, no matter how loudly my family shouted for me. I have done lots of silly things during my triathlon adventures, but resolutely refusing to race, and locking myself in a filthy toilet to hide, must be the most ridiculous and embarrassing.

I began the day with the best of intentions.

I had been on a post-triathlon high for about a week after completing that first race in Chester. I had loved the experience, even if I did have to overcome nausea-inducing nerves beforehand, freezing cold fingers and feet while cycling, stumbling through the run and the unsettling panic in the swim. All that dissolved into memory as soon as I crossed the finish line; all I could think about was how much fun it had been to be racing. And when I saw my results, I was delighted: it turned out, I was quite good at something I enjoyed.

I had well and truly caught the triathlon bug. I would have to do another one.

After tackling my fear of murky water in the River Dee 5 kilometres, I signed up to do a supersprint triathlon organised by the Olympic medal-winning brothers Alistair and Jonathan Brownlee. Supersprint just means that the distances are much shorter – and should, of course, mean that you are able to go faster.

The setting was stunning. Fountains Abbey is a ruined Cistercian monastery, founded in 1123 and now a UNESCO World Heritage Site. It has a beautiful Georgian water garden, complete with ponds, statues and follies, all surrounded by a medieval deer park that is home to red, fallow and sika deer.

The 400-metre swim in Studley Royal Lake would be followed by a 10-kilometre bike ride through the park and then a 2.5-kilometre run through Studley Royal Water Garden, the final sprint taking us on a blue carpet through the ruins of the Abbey itself. It was an incredibly dramatic setting.

The only slight problem was the timing. I was due to present *BBC Breakfast* that day, so I would have to do the triathlon after four hours of presenting the programme and a considerable drive. I worked out that it was about a two-hour drive from MediaCity in Salford Quays to Ripon. If we left at 10 o'clock after the programme had finished, this would give me just about enough time to get there, stack all my gear in transition, and join my race wave. With David driving, this would also mean, all things being well, I might be able to sneak in a bit of a snooze in the car.

The night before, I got all my kit ready, packed it into the car and hoped that I had remembered everything. I was quite calm about the whole thing, thinking that I was perfectly capable of pulling off a day's work and a race – right up until David, the girls and Waffle arrived to pick me up about half an hour late.

Half an hour late! I couldn't believe it, and then came a panic of epic proportions. I was huffing, puffing, and chuntering about how we weren't going to get there, that we might as well go straight home and give up right now. I was beside myself.

In reply, they were all, quite rightly, telling me to stop being so silly and to calm down, insisting that of course we were going to make it. I had almost decided to believe them, and had calmed down a touch, when we drove straight into a long traffic jam. When I saw the line of cars stretching before us, any idea of having a restful snooze went right out of the window – exactly like my sense of humour!

By the time we eventually arrived at Fountains Abbey, I had indeed missed my wave. I was so cross that effectively I went on strike. I refused point-blank to get ready for the race: as far as I was concerned, I had missed my slot, which meant it was game over. We might as well turn around and head home.

Having been cooped up in the car for hours, David, Mia, Scarlett and probably Waffle the dog, too, were furious with me. I had made them get up early in the morning, drive for miles and now we had arrived, they couldn't believe that I was refusing even to get into my wetsuit.

While I moaned on about how hopeless the situation was, they went to check with the race organisers if it would be possible for me to start in another, later wave. It was, and they gave me no choice, tipping my stuff out of the car, marching me to registration, making me glue on my race numbers, and then depositing me and my bike in transition.

Behaving as badly as a spoilt child, and at the same time pretending I was getting my kit ready, I was still muttering away to myself. *Why am I bothering, it's all pointless, and why am I doing this anyway?* Despite the effort of getting there, all the preparation and the fact that I had inconvenienced my whole family by making them wake up in the early hours of a Saturday morning, I was adamant: I didn't want to race. I decided to make sure I didn't get to the start.

That's how I ended up in the Portaloo.

My family knew I would try to take evasive action, and were keeping a close eye on me. Even so, I saw an opportunity to escape, sneaked out of transition, flounced off and locked myself in the loo. From inside my unhygienic sanctuary, I could hear them calling for me, but I stayed exactly where I was, not planning to come out.

Mia, who has as much determination as I do, eventually found me and started pounding on the door. 'Come on, Mummy! For goodness' sake, just get in the water, it's nearly the last wave! You're going to miss it altogether.'

Shamed for my childish behaviour by a 12-year-old, I pulled myself together. Mustering some determination, I sheepishly came out, and lied as convincingly as I could. 'Sorry, I was just having a bit of a problem with my zip, thanks for coming to get me.' Mia then marched me to the start, with David and Scarlett acting as close escort.

As soon as I hit the water, it was all, miraculously, OK. I managed to get out right at the front and set off at a calm but fast pace. The 5-kilometre big swim in the river had made a massive difference. Although there were weeds pulling at my feet and face, I just didn't care, sliding through the water with huge confidence, easily navigating round the large orange buoys and back to the start. I came out of the water laughing, with a huge grin on my face, to be greeted by Waffle, who had escaped her lead and was leaping about and barking excitedly.

The bike ride was speedy too, out through the stunning deer park in a double loop. Apart from one long Yorkshire hill, I whizzed along, loving every minute. Even the run wasn't as bad as I had expected, and I managed to overtake a couple of people as I jogged along the side of the lake and through the elegant and peaceful Studley Royal Water Garden.

The final sprint was spectacular. Running right through the middle of the Abbey's dramatic ruins, I was neck and neck with another competitor as we hit the traditional triathlon blue carpet laid out along the nave. Although I didn't beat him to the line, I was thrilled to finish the race – especially as I had tried my absolute best not to even start it.

Post-race celebrations that day were made by meeting and taking a celebration photograph with both the Brownlee brothers, and then watching as they tumbled over each other on a huge inflatable assault course.

My results took a while to come through. I had confused the computer system by missing my wave, so the first set of results recorded my swim-time as over an hour. When my actual start time was calculated, the final result showed that I had completed the 400-metre swim in 6.58, which made me very proud; the bike in 25.24; and the run in a more pedestrian 14.17.

The day had started off terribly, and it was only thanks to the persistence and encouragement of my family that I had even dipped my toe in the water. If it were not for them, I would have failed even to try. When I finished my race, I was profoundly apologetic and grateful, and treated them to a round of cakes and ice creams in the café to make up for my behaviour. Thankfully, and because I had actually raced, they did forgive me. Otherwise, they would never have let me live it down. Shame, it turns out, is a forceful motivator!

I went home tired but elated and determined never to let nerves overcome me again and make me behave like a spoilt child.

My final result was an added incentive: this time around, even after all those pre-race shenanigans, I had managed to come fourth in my age group.

I was moving up the rankings.

CHAPTER 7

DEMORALISED AND DESTABILISED

'The point when triathlon became more than a sport I did for a bit of occasional fun.'

A few months after those first, exhilarating forays into the world of triathlon, I hit a surprisingly difficult period in my working life. This had a profound effect on my approach to sport, and my motivation for doing it – and, bizarrely, it was all to do with *Strictly Come Dancing*.

Since April 2012, when *Breakfast* had moved from BBC Television Centre in London to MediaCity in Salford, Susanna Reid and I had been sharing presenting duties on the programme.

Susanna had been presenting the first half of the week – Monday, Tuesday and Wednesday – alongside Bill Turnbull, and Charlie Stayt and myself presented the other half of the week – Thursday, Friday and Saturday. Since moving location, we had been a happy team: our viewing figures continued to be excellent, with more than six and a half million people watching every day, and we were consistently beating our rivals on *Daybreak*.

The arrangement with Susanna and I splitting the week worked well, until she signed up to be part of the *Strictly* cast in the run-up to Christmas 2013. For her to be able to take part, Adam Bullimore, the editor of *BBC Breakfast*, asked me if I would also present Mondays. I was very happy to say yes.

Susanna, who had won the newsreaders' *BBC Children in Need 'Strictly Come Dancing Special'*, did brilliantly in the Saturday night competition, wowing both the judges and the public with her fantastic, dynamic partnership with Kevin Clifton. They stormed through week after week, and went all the way to the final, where they eventually lost out on the glitter ball to model Abbey Clancy.

Her huge success on *Strictly* meant that by Christmas 2013, Susanna and her future career were front-page news. There were reports that ITV was wooing her, offering her a huge salary to tempt her to leave the BBC.

In March, the news broke that she had decided to resign. It was devastating to hear that she was indeed going to leave behind what had been a happy and successful team, but then we had to absorb the news that she had been poached to present a brand new breakfast programme called *Good Morning Britain*.

What followed was an unedifying flurry of newspaper speculation about who was going to replace her on *BBC Breakfast*. All sorts of names were bandied about, including Sky's stalwart presenter Kay Burley, *Countdown*'s numbers guru Rachel Riley, *Daybreak*'s Christine Bleakley and *Breakfast*'s weather presenter, Carol Kirkwood.

What was immediately obvious was that, even though Susanna had already left, the BBC were in no hurry to decide how, or even if, they were going to replace her.

That left me in a tricky position.

Someone had to present the programme while a choice was made, and the person they asked was me. This was great, of course, but it was made clear there would be no guarantee that I would continue presenting the front end of the week. The management were actively looking for, interviewing and screen-testing other people.

In that febrile atmosphere, my confidence took a blow. I began to feel that every day I was presenting the programme was an audition for the job. I began to worry that if I got even a tiny thing wrong, made a mistake or an unforced error, my future at *Breakfast* would disintegrate. It was demoralising and destabilising.

To avoid being brought down, I decided I would have to put my heart and soul into something else. I needed a distraction from feeling I had no control over my own destiny.

That was a pivotal moment for me, and the point when triathlon became more than a sport I did for a bit of occasional fun. It had already brought me a huge sense of achievement, but now it became more than that; it became a safe haven. Whenever I was swimming, running or cycling, I wasn't worrying about what was going on at work or what the future might hold. I was just doing something I loved – and enjoying the moment.

The splash of cold water on my face diving into a lake at the start of an open-water swim. Stopping my bike for a minute on a bridge over the river, and catching sight of a heron standing tall on a fallen branch, waiting patiently for a passing fish. Watching Waffle jogging contentedly through the puddles beside me as we ran through another freezing rain shower. There were so many moments like that, and I enjoyed every single one of them. Together they made a difference to my sense of well-being.

Sport became a wonderful and welcome escape.

The training had its everyday benefits, but in triathlon I had also found a place where I could compete on an even playing field.

Any success I achieved had a direct correlation not just to ability but to the work and effort I made. If I put in the hours running, swimming or cycling, I would get faster. It didn't matter what I looked like, I would be judged only on the hard facts, seconds and minutes. It was a revelation, empowering me and helping massively with my sporting motivation.

That spring and summer went by in a blur of exercise. I began to train four or five times a week, swimming, running or cycling, depending on my mood, and I started to absolutely love it. To help with organisation and motivation, I took on a new coach and set myself different sporting goals.

I completed another 5-kilometre swim, this time in the pool at Olympic Park in Stratford for *Sport Relief*, and I ran the Great Manchester 10k Run, managing to finish under the hour, in just over 56 minutes.

David and I even entered – and completed – a three-day, 300-mile bike ride from Cornwall to London. We signed up for the Milligan Bike Ride, staged in memory of our dear friend Nicko Milligan and his eight-year-old daughter Emily, who were killed in a tragic speedboat accident in Padstow, Cornwall. More than a hundred cyclists rode together, to raise money for the Royal National Lifeboat Institution (RNLI) and Child Bereavement UK. It was by far the toughest thing either of us had ever done, with back-breaking hills, 14 hours a day in the saddle and floods of tears at the finish line.

I also went back to the Brownlee Tri for a second time. This time I didn't lock myself in the loo in a nervous panic at the start, and I loved the race.

Eventually in July 2014, four months after Susanna had left and six months after the speculation about her replacement began, the BBC announced that Naga Munchetty had been chosen to join the *Breakfast* team full-time. The good news for me was that I would continue presenting at the beginning of the week, as I had been since Susanna's departure.

I was delighted they had chosen Naga. She is a talented and experienced presenter, and an excellent journalist. And having presented on Sundays regularly for years, she was already part of the *BBC Breakfast* family.

Those six months of uncertainty had been tough, and it was sport that had pulled me through. Distracting me from my energy-sapping worry, it got me exercising almost every single day, and gave me a massive sense of achievement every time I finished a hard training session.

My triathlon training had started as a sideshow to help me cope with anxiety, but now it had taken on a life of its own. It was a passion, an integral part of my life, and I was at the start of a sporting adventure.

I was hooked. There was no way I was going to give it up.

CHAPTER 8

REPRESENT GREAT BRITAIN? SERIOUSLY?

'You were internally 100 per cent committed to achieving it. Eighty per cent was not enough.'

Claire Sutcliffe, triathlon coach

At some time in my second year of competing, with seven or eight different races and events to my name, a friend made a chance remark. 'You are doing incredibly well. Do you know, if you get a qualifying time in a qualifying triathlon, you can compete for Great Britain in your age group in the World Championships or the European Championships?'

I couldn't believe it. Me, competing in the World or European Championships? Really? What a ridiculous idea! How can a 46-year-old, long-term resident of the *BBC Breakfast* red sofa get up and represent her country in a sport she took up only two years ago? How utterly absurd, and how totally brilliant! What an honour it would be, I thought, to wear a tri suit carrying the Union Flag!

An incredible idea, but could I possibly do it? How tough and challenging would it be? And did I have the slightest chance of even being close?

Once the idea was planted in my head, it wouldn't go away. I remembered all those times when the people competing alongside me were proudly wearing their red, white and blue Great Britain suits. I had often wondered how they managed to get them, and now I knew. They were what are referred to in the triathlon world as 'age-groupers', representing the UK in their age group against triathletes from all over the world. How awesome and inspirational was that?

The thought took hold and kept nagging at me. Was I fast enough in one of the disciplines, let alone all three? Was it far too ambitious? Was it too hard to even try?

To answer these questions, I turned to my coach, Claire Sutcliffe, with whom I had been working for about a year.

I first met Claire at an exercise class she ran for some of the mothers from my daughter's school. The Mums' Boot Camp consisted of running around the park in Chester, followed by some strenuous strength and conditioning exercises. I liked Claire right from the start. She had a no-nonsense, tough but positive approach, which I found very motivating. When I discovered that she was a very successful triathlete in her own right and that she also coached triathletes, I asked if she would help me too.

She is a fantastic coach, incredibly organised and with a wonderful ability to be firm but encouraging at the same time. In the year or so she had been coaching me, her training plans had steered me through several triathlons, the Manchester 10k Run, and the 5-kilometre swim for *Sport Relief*.

Even so, I didn't dare tell her what my next challenge might be, mainly because I thought she would tell me I was bonkers.

Instead, I had a peek at the British Triathlon website and found that there were three qualifiers a year for the World Championships and three for the European Championships. To be successful I would have to compete in at least a couple of them, and the countdown had already begun. The first was in a mere eight months' time.

I had so many questions, and the only person who could answer them was Claire. I knew that if anyone could help get me to the World Championships it would be her, but I was reluctant to ask. I feared it would be several steps too far for me.

Much to my surprise, when I told her she was thrilled. 'Yes, that's a brilliant idea, let's do this.'

Her thoughts then turned to the practicalities of trying to qualify. She was brutally honest, and told me that I couldn't possibly be at the top of my age group: I had been in the sport for only 18 months, and it would be physically impossible to knock large enough chunks of time off every discipline. But if I was 100 per cent committed, if I focused on each sport individually, if I put in hours of hard work and training – then, all being well, I might get to a point where I secured a qualifying time.

It was going to be tough.

Then she broke the daunting news: to have any chance at all, I was going to have to double the distance that I had raced so far.

In the short period of time we had before the crucial races, I was never going to be fast enough to be able to qualify in the sprint distance races. The 5-kilometre run times in my age group effectively ruled me out. So far, my fastest 5 kilometres had been over 25 minutes, and most of my age group in the Great Britain team were running very close to, or often under, 20 minutes. Both my bike and swim times would also have to be considerably faster.

She reckoned my best option would be to try to qualify for what is called 'Standard' or 'Olympic' distance triathlon. That is the distance raced by Jonathan and Alistair Brownlee at the Olympics.

I had never raced that far before, and it meant that I would have to double the distance in each of the three disciplines. The swim would now be 1,500 metres, the bike 40 kilometres and the run 10 kilometres. I already found half the distance tough to race, so this was daunting, especially the run. In my training, I routinely never ran more than about seven kilometres – and even that was a struggle. So just the thought of cycling for more than an hour and then trying to finish a 10-kilometre run was exhausting. How was I going to manage it?

Claire also took me through British Triathlon rules about qualification. They are a little bit complicated, but sort of fascinating – especially for a triathlon nerd like me – so bear with me. I will try and make it fun!

There are normally four qualification places available in each age group for each of the three qualifying races, twelve automatic spaces in total. These are given out in descending order to the triathletes who have registered their interest in qualifying. So, if you come first out of the registered athletes in a qualifying race, you get the first qualifying place. That means a prestigious Q1 by your name on the British Triathlon website. You don't necessarily have to be first in your race to get the Q1, because the athletes who beat you might not have registered to qualify.

Are you with me so far?

Good; it goes on. If you don't get one of those automatic slots, there is then a roll-down system for the remaining eight places.

Every triathlon course is different and so, to make it fair across the three qualifiers, British Triathlon compare your race finish time to that of the winner in your age group and give you a percentage of their time. You will be considered for a roll-down slot only if your time is within 115 per cent of the winning time in your age group. The closer your percentage is to the winner's time, the higher up you are on the list. Simple!

The significance of all the above will become obvious later.

Now, back to the training!

The alarming scale of what I was going to have to do soon became obvious. Claire checked the winning times in my age group for the Deva Triathlon in Chester, which had been a World Championship Qualifier the year before, in 2014. This gave us a useful benchmark to judge my performance: I had done the bike leg of the same triathlon as part of a relay team in 2014, and had finished the 40 kilometres in 1 hour, 24 minutes. When we looked at the results, we could see that my bike time was a full 10 minutes slower than the top five women in my age group, who had also done the swim and the run. Ten minutes!

Their run times were even more impressive: the winner, Karen Bridge, had clocked a super speedy 43 minutes, 12 seconds. My fastest 10 kilometres, not in a triathlon, was a whopping 56 minutes! A difference of 13 minutes!

The only upside was this: my run was so slow compared to everyone else, there was lots of room for improvement.

My swimming speeds were my one advantage. From what we knew about my open-water races so far, my pace meant I should be somewhere close to the best swimmers, and faster than most of the rest of the field.

Even so, the raw numbers made it quite clear that I had a mountain to climb.

I wasn't convinced I could manage it, but Claire was.

'I thought you could do it because of your personality. If you want something, and say you are going to do it, you will be able to do it. Even if you wouldn't say it aloud, deep down you were determined enough to know you could do it, and crucially you believed you could do it. Some people say they want to do it, but as a coach you know they are not focused enough to hit all those main sessions. You were internally 100 per cent committed to achieving it. Eighty per cent was not enough.'

The night of our discussion Claire sent me an email detailing what I had to do in each discipline. There was no time for slacking. Training began straightaway, six days a week.

CHAPTER 9

MARGINAL GAINS

'I was still embarrassed by the memory of being called Ozzie the Ostrich by one of my friends at university, because of my inelegant running gait.'

If I wanted to make it into the team, there was no time to lose. There is a lot of talk in sport about 'marginal gains'. Used by the likes of British Cycling, the term describes how making a lot of small or marginal differences can lead to big improvements or gains in your overall time. My gains were going to have to be a good deal more than marginal, though. They would have to be huge!

Claire and I had our initial conversation at the end of October, and I would have to be race-ready by June.

To make the significant improvements needed to get my hands on a GB suit, I faced eight months of hard effort, training for an hour and a half, six or seven days a week; two swims, three runs and two bike rides, every week for 30 weeks. I would have to fit that around getting up in the early hours to present *Breakfast*, and a busy life as a mum.

And as if the amount of time I was going to have to put in were not intimidating enough, I also had to radically improve my technique for everything: swimming, cycling and running.

The priority was my cycling.

I loved it, but wasn't nearly fast or strong enough.

To speed up, I needed to get in some serious miles. Winter was approaching, so rather than be out in the dark on the wet or icy roads, the best way to improve was to get hold of a turbo trainer.

I thought a turbo was a type of engine that makes your car go faster. In fact, in cycling terms it is a large metal A-frame with a heavy wheel on the back, which acts as a roller. You put the back wheel of your road bike on it, back the tyre up against the roller, adjust the resistance with your gears and then start pedalling while your bike is semi-suspended. It means that you can ride your road bike and train while you are stationary and, more importantly, indoors – cosy and safe.

I didn't have a turbo, but was kindly lent one by Matt Dimbylow, a GB Paralympic footballer and a friend. He showed me how to set it up and how to balance (precariously!) on it – and warned me it would be hard work. He was right, it was. But it was also an effective way of training in the comfort of my own home, rather than out in the rain or on icy roads, cowering away from cars and lorries.

Once I knew how to work it, I sat pedalling like a lunatic, in the surroundings of my own kitchen, completing the increasingly tough sessions that Claire had set me. Much to the hilarity of David and the girls, I would dismount about an hour later, looking as if I had just stepped out of a shower, I was so sweaty.

Running was a much bigger problem than cycling, but it was the sport where I could potentially make some significant progress. I had an ongoing, niggly pain in my foot – and the more I ran, the more it hurt.

Claire had a plan. She needed me to be running 8–9 miles regularly with no pain. Once I could get to that distance, then we could start doing some speed work. To do that she recommended I start going to the gym to do some weight training, and concentrate on strength and conditioning.

Claire also suggested that I start running with the Chester Triathlon Club at the local athletics track. What a terrifying thought! I had never stepped on to an athletics track, not even at school. Why would I want to do that now?

In my imagination, the triathlon track session would be full of super-fit runners, who would laugh at my ungainly running style. I was still embarrassed by the memory of being called Ozzie the Ostrich by one of my friends at university, because of my inelegant running gait. I imagined he was referring to my long legs, knobbly knees and big, sticking-out bottom! Whatever it was, I had never forgotten it, and still felt ashamed of my running.

It took me ages to pluck up courage to go to the running club, making every imaginable excuse possible not to go. Eventually I forced myself to drive there, on a rainy Wednesday night in January, to join a cross section of runners warming up by gently jogging round the track. They could not have been more welcoming. I quickly learned what seemed to be the first essential rule of track etiquette: if you aren't running, get off the track and out of the way!

I had thought I would be by far the slowest – and I was. But nobody laughed at me. Instead, they were incredibly supportive. The two coaches, Dave Taylor and Kelly Crickmore, dutifully recorded my times, and even when I was lapped whoever lapped me would shout encouragement.

I also had to get miles under my belt. To make any improvement, I needed to be running at least three times a week. Claire had prescribed a mixture of different types of runs: some of them with faster pace work; others including some hills; and longer, slower, endurance runs.

I dreaded the running, but luckily there is someone in my house who thinks it is the best thing in the world: Waffle. She is an incredibly loyal, enthusiastic running companion, eager to get out whatever the weather and help motivate me along the way.

As for swimming, that was likely to be by far my best discipline. Even so, I couldn't rest on my laurels.

Every second I could save on my swim would take me a second closer to getting into the team. So, if possible, I had to swim faster too. More importantly, every second I managed to gain in the swim was one I didn't have to worry about on the run – a useful psychological boost.

To make any significant difference, though, I needed to improve on my technique.

I can't count how many times people say to me, *I would love to do triathlon but I am not a good swimmer*, or *I hate swimming*. I have a standard reply: Whatever your standard is in swimming, you can always improve. Even though I can swim well, I still have lessons on technique.

My first stop on the swimming improvement plan was to visit a startlingly unglamorous location: an industrial unit round the back of a business park in Chester.

I was genuinely scared when I arrived and caught my first glimpse of it on a cold February morning. It reminded me of a run-down, spine-chilling location from *Silent Witness*, and looked like a particularly inauspicious place to go for a swim.

When I dared to get out of my car and open the creaking metal door, what I found was a crystal-clear pool about 3 metres long by 2 metres wide. The pool had a flume at one end, which pumped out a stream of water at varying speeds. So, once you were brave enough to get in it, you could swim against the current.

The genius of this pool was that it had cameras above the water and under the water. This meant that Chris Malpass, the coach behind the appropriately named company U Can Swim, could film my swimming stroke and give me some instant analysis.

It was quickly obvious that I had two issues.

First, I kept my arm straight underwater, which meant I was only using my weaker muscles, and wasting lots of energy. Second, I didn't breathe properly. The recording showed clearly that I took a breath only once I had turned my head so far that I was looking at the ceiling – which not only wasted time but meant my whole stroke was off balance. If I made a couple of adjustments, Chris told me, my stroke rate would slow down but I would be going faster.

With all the different elements to concentrate on, I had an incredible amount of work to do. It was exhausting, and frustrating because the rewards would not be immediate. Any gain was only going to be incremental; nothing would improve dramatically overnight. But I was determined. I knuckled down and did my absolute best to follow Claire's training plan.

Whatever the weather, I would force myself to get outside and drive my unwilling legs on cold, wet training runs accompanied by Waffle. I would sacrifice a lie-in and get up early on a Saturday to immerse myself in the pool for an early morning technique session. And I would drive the girls nuts sweating away on the turbo in the kitchen, breathlessly interrupting their television viewing.

I was utterly determined that I would knuckle down, put in the hours, ignore the pain, deal with the exhaustion, and commit as much time and energy as I could to Claire's training plan.

It would be months before I could judge whether all the effort would be worth it.

CHAPTER 10

COLD, TIRED BUT DETERMINED

'Why don't I just stop being so silly, quit running, walk back and have a nice cup of tea and a cake with my family?'

There are so many things I love about triathlon. One is that you cannot do the sport unless you are a trier – by which I mean that you must have an absolute determination to do the best you can whatever happens. It is just too complicated and challenging to be someone who gives up when things big or small go wrong – and my goodness, they do go wrong!

I have completed some classic triathlons: some hurt on the day, some hurt for months, and some still make me laugh every time I think about them.

One of the most challenging triathlons I have ever done was in Machynlleth, a beautiful market town in the Dyfi Valley, Wales.

We were inspired by one of our close friends, Ian Blandford, who had been signed up by his wife and great friend of ours, Jay Hunt, to do the triathlon in the town as a birthday present. Over a New Year's dinner and more than a glass or two of wine, David and I thought it would be a good idea to sign up too. We could race alongside each other. David had never done a triathlon and was very apprehensive, especially to be competing against his friend and his wife. He knew he would be lucky to beat either of us.

Ian, who is a keen mountain biker, was by far the fittest of us all. He had been a competitive triathlete some 15 years ago but hadn't completed one since. I knew I would probably beat him on the swim, but he would be much faster than either of us on both the bike and the run.

Over what seemed like a short couple of months between that alcohol-influenced decision to race and the actual triathlon, David and I trained together, getting out on our bikes once a week when I got home from *Breakfast* and running regularly with Waffle. He is a good swimmer, but he isn't very confident, so I coached him in the pool as well. He started to speed up and feel more comfortable in the water.

I wouldn't claim that either of us were at peak fitness on the day of the race. We were both nervous, but were also really looking forward to it. As we headed west from our home in Chester to Mid Wales in the early morning, the clouds descended along with the temperature. The skies darkened – and so did our mood as we watched the windscreen wipers work overtime sweeping sleet off the glass.

It was going to be a difficult race for us all.

Things started going wrong as soon as I got my bike out of the car. In the early hours of the morning we had taken the bikes apart to fit them both in the car, and as we were reassembling mine, the bracket holding the stem of my seat in place snapped. What a disaster! I couldn't ride 20 kilometres without a seat. This had never happened before and we had no idea what to do, nor any suitable equipment to fix it.

Slightly panicky and with dozens of people also rushing around having pre-race jitters, I asked one of the race volunteers if he could come up with anything. Unbelievably, even though he was riding on a mountain bike and mine was a road bike, the bracket for his seat was a perfect match for mine. Very generously, he took it off and fixed my bike so that I could race.

In my panic I then also managed to lose my Garmin watch, which was like a race lifeline for me. Without it, I would have no idea how fast or slow I was going and, more importantly, how much effort I needed to make.

After the shenanigans with the broken bike, we just about got all our gear into transition in time. By then, it was pouring with rain and it was also very cold. I was delighted to see that David and I had consecutive race numbers. This meant our bike stations were positioned right opposite each other on the gravel in the car park, meaning that we could check and double-check our equipment together: bikes, helmets, new bike shoes, trainers, and some food and drink.

We then had a quick look at how to get in and out of the transition area before we went into the steamy swimming pool complex. I would much prefer to race in open water, but given the appalling weather, I was very grateful that the swim was in an indoor pool. The pool had only four or five lanes and there were about a hundred of us competing, so it meant we would have to wait poolside for some time for others to finish their swim before we could start.

Two people swam in each lane, and when one competitor finished, another would jump in, a bit like a mass relay. It was a 400-metre swim in a 20-metre pool, so 20 lengths for each of us.

While we waited, fidgety and twitchy with pre-race nerves, we sat on the floor leaning back against the wall and chatting as we watched a partially sighted woman being guided through her swim by her daughter, who was walking up and down along the edge of the pool, telling her when to turn and where to swim. The woman was the first leg of a relay team, and when she finished and hauled herself out of the water, all the waiting triathletes gave her a huge cheer as she handed over the baton to her daughter, who did the bike leg of the race.

Alongside her were several people of all different ages swimming in GB triathlon suits. I was impressed by how fast some of them were in the water, and also daunted – this was the level I was hoping to reach. I hate the waiting at the start of a race: I just want to get on with it, and watching others only makes me even more nervous.

In our group of three, Ian was due to start about 20 minutes before us. We watched him push himself hard, up and down the pool. He managed a fast swim and leapt out of the pool with a big grin on his face, super-confident. In his haste to get to his bike, he ran beside the pool – disobeying the rules and earning himself a telling-off from an official.

David and I were going to be among the last few to start, and we had hatched a plan of sorts so that we could at least begin the cycle section together.

We knew that I was likely to be quicker than him in the pool, so he went first, to start his swim a couple of minutes ahead of me. Assuming I did manage to catch him up, that meant we would be in transition together, making the process much more enjoyable, and allowing us to set off on the bike course in tandem.

David hates swimming, and he had been dreading it, but my coaching seemed to pay off. I was delighted to see him set off at a good pace and successfully negotiate his first turn.

Then it was my turn to sit on the edge of the pool and adjust my goggles. I listened carefully to the race organiser, who explained that when I had reached the last two lengths they would let me know it was time to stop by tapping me on the head with a pool buoy. The water felt stiflingly hot, and it seemed bizarre to be swimming under the children's waterslide, which swooped over our heads into the deep end.

This was only a 20-metre pool and I had been training in a 25-metre pool, so the end of each length arrived much sooner than I imagined it would. It wasn't long before I felt the tap on my head, which meant there were just two more lengths to go before it was time to drag myself out. I couldn't see how David was doing but, just as we had hoped, I came out of the pool moments after him and followed closely in the trail of his wet footsteps.

I was wearing my wet tri suit and my hair was sopping, and the icy blast of air in the car park knocked the breath out of me. I was instantly frozen, but so pleased to be in transition at the same time as David. We both laughed at the madness of what we were doing, sitting on the ground in a car park in the freezing cold, wearing sodden clothes and rushing to get our bike shoes on.

Mine were brand new, all neatly laid out and with the fastenings done up. Here came Challenge No. 2: my fingers were numb and, try as I might, I couldn't work out how to undo them so that I could put them on my now frozen feet. I was losing precious seconds in the race.

My saviour, David, who can get me out of most scrapes, also had a go – but even he couldn't work out what was wrong with them and why we couldn't undo the buckles. A race volunteer could see us struggling and had a try too, but it was hopeless. None of us could budge the fastenings and there was no way I could squeeze them on to my feet without undoing them. What on earth was I going to do? The pedals on my bike aren't designed to be used with any other shoes but I was going to have to do just that: cycle with my trainers perched on top of the narrow metal clips and hope that it worked.

In my agitation, I shoved on my helmet, did it up, and was about to get on my bike when a race official started shouting at me, 'Helmet, helmet!'

I had no idea what he was talking about, and he had to shout louder before I realised that I had put my helmet on back to front. I swapped it around as quickly as I could and thought I had got away with it, but the very quick race photographer managed to get a hilarious picture of me looking very uncool with my helmet perched back to front.

After the shoe shambles, I set off at a cracking pace, trying my hardest to make sure the double whammy of the shoe and helmet incident would make no difference to my time. I passed David on the first turn, thinking he would catch me on the bike. And if, somehow, he didn't, there was no doubt that he would overtake me in the run.

It was a brutal bike ride, heading out of Machynlleth into a blasting wind, but my trainers seemed to be working and the extra impetus of wasting time made me more determined to try and catch some of the cyclists out in front. I was looking out for Ian, but he had started 20 minutes before us in the pool, and must have set off at a cracking pace because I never caught sight of him at all. After pushing hard up three or four leg-sapping inclines, I made the 10-kilometre turnaround and realised I must have been going quite fast, as David still hadn't passed me. I caught a glimpse of him as I came flying down one of the long hills, and gave him a manic grin and a wave.

Not having my bike shoes on did offer a brilliant advantage: when I came to transition, all I had to do was throw my bike on to the metal bike rack and sprint. Excellent, but in my haste, I had another helmet disaster. I was so paranoid about breaking the rules and not touching my helmet until my bike was racked that I dashed on to the run leg still wearing my helmet. At a qualifying race for the World or European Championships, you would have to take it off, run back and put it with your bike – and yes, I have done that, too! But the race volunteers let me leave it on the ground, and run on. I say 'leave it', but the race photographer told me later that, in my hurry, I threw it on the ground and nearly hit him with it.

I always find the running the hardest discipline, and when I looked down to see hail bouncing off my fists as I tackled the first hill, I had one of those many moments in triathlon when the negative thoughts start to bite:

What on earth am I doing? I must be utterly mad to be out in the freezing cold, dragging my heavy legs on a 5-kilometre run. Why don't I just stop being so silly, quit running, walk back and have a nice cup of tea and a cake with my family?

It's at these moments, when I think I have hit rock bottom, that some magic and powerful extra gear sets in. I thought: *I am not going to give up now! If I do, I am letting myself and everyone else down.* I put my head down and forced myself to concentrate on putting one foot in front of the other to push through the gloom.

The weather was bitterly cold with the cloud enveloping the tops of the surrounding hills, but the views of the wild Welsh countryside were stunning. We ran past sheep still grazing and ignoring the sleet, over cattle grids and a golf course, all of which served to distract me from the cold.

As I reached the top of the last hill, I looked back to see David about half a mile behind me, catching me up fast. That was enough to reignite my sense of competition: I wasn't going to let him catch me at this late stage! He had seen me, too, and thought he could easily make up the distance between us. In training, and especially in a sprint, he is much faster than me – but no, not this time. It was a total surprise to both of us that I found an extra burst of speed, scooting around the last couple of corners, back to the Leisure Centre and straight into the arms of my patient but frozen daughters, who were trying to hold back Waffle, who was straining to get off her lead.

I still hadn't caught my breath when David finished a couple of minutes behind me. He gave me a huge sweaty hug, despite his frustration at being beaten by his wife. We were exhausted but elated to have finished.

There was still no sign of Ian, and we were worried. Where had he gone? We knew that he would have finished far ahead of us, but we expected him to be there laughing at us and lapping up the glory.

We caught sight of him wrapped in a first-aid foil sheet, shaking and extremely pale. He limped towards us. He had raced so fast that he had nearly collapsed on the finish line, and had gone into spasms of uncontrollable shaking. By the time we saw him, he had the shakes under control, but he was still shivering and was monosyllabic. It was alarmingly unlike him. When the going gets tough, he is always the one who cajoles us into carrying on, so to see him in such a state was worrying. His family were clearly concerned too, but had waited to see if we were both OK before they bundled him into the car to take him back home and warm him up in a hot bath.

We followed shortly afterwards, gathering up our bikes and assorted belongings, putting on some dry clothes, turning up the car heater to maximum and heading off to meet them for lunch. By the time we got to the restaurant in the centre of town, Ian was – thank goodness – warm and cheery again, back to his gregarious self and with a pint in his hand. After large portions of risotto and roast beef, we too made fast recoveries. And all of us, including the now less frozen spectators, were laughing at the sheer lunacy of the day.

It might have been a tough race, but it was also fantastic fun. We had all taken part in an amazing adventure together, and would have both good and bad memories. Ian had raced extremely well, beating me by a whole 10 minutes, but David and I could go home proud in the knowledge that we had come fourth and fifth in our age groups.

The extreme challenges of that race still serve me well.

If I'm at a competition and finding it difficult, I just picture myself running in soaking wet clothes in the freezing cold and with hail bouncing off my hands and think, *Well, it's not as tough as that, so just get a flipping move on.* I also always check that my bike shoes are undone, and will never put my helmet on back to front again.

Since then, neither David nor Ian have completed another triathlon! That bitterly frozen day was enough for them – and I totally understand why. On the other hand, I was even more determined to qualify as a Great Britain triathlete.

CHAPTER 11

LEARNING AND IMPROVING

'After two hours of a gold-medal winning athlete shouting instructions at me, I felt broken.'

Eight months had now passed since that first conversation with Claire. Eight months since admitting my madly ambitious dream of getting into the Great Britain triathlon team. During those winter months, I had tried hard to train as much as possible. Predictably, though, not everything went to plan.

In an ideal world, Claire wanted me at the point where I could run about 10 miles comfortably. The reality was, I achieved only about four miles before my injured foot started playing up. It was seriously painful, and it was obvious that the running was the issue. My physiotherapist had given me more exercises to try to strengthen it, but it was clear that there was no quick fix or miracle cure, and I was struggling to know what to do. Unexpectedly, I had a lucky break.

I was asked by Channel 4 to take part in what was described as a living history programme, *Time Crashers*. The premise was that a group of celebrities would be taken back in time to live, as realistically as possible, in different eras of British history – everything from Tudor to Victorian England and all the way back to the Iron Age.

At the outset, it looked like committing to the three-week filming schedule would be a hindrance rather than a help for my training plan; there were obviously no bicycles or swimming pools in most of the historical periods we would be living in. As it turned out, though, there was a very surprising upside. When I signed up for the programme, what I didn't know was that Olympic gold medal-winning long jumper Greg Rutherford would also be taking part.

Right at the start of filming, while Greg was gutting chickens dressed in a Tudor tunic and I was dressed up as a maid washing clothes in urine – as they did in the 15th century – we had a conversation about sport, triathlon and injury. I told him about what I was trying to do, and he promised that on the next break we had from filming, he would look at my running and see if there was something I might be able to do to improve it.

He was true to his word. When we had some time off, he made me, *Coronation Street* actor Charlie Condou and GB Commonwealth gold-winning weightlifter Zoe Smith train with him. He worked us incredibly hard, copying him in a series of exercises that his coaches had given him specifically to strengthen his running. We were skipping, hopping, running backwards, sideways, and then repeatedly up and down a steep hill at maximum effort. The session was so challenging that after the last sprint up the incline I was nearly sick. Greg just laughed. After two hours of a gold-medal winning athlete shouting instructions at me, I felt broken.

Greg also looked very carefully at my running gait, and taught me how to plant my foot in a way that would make it much more stable, and hopefully stop exacerbating my injury.

What an incredibly lucky break for me! It was exactly what I needed to improve my running.

When I left *Time Crashers*, I continued with the exercises and worked hard on concentrating and trying to correct my running gait. The good news was that my foot stopped hurting so much – and I started running a bit more like an athlete and less like a giraffe.

I felt much better, but I didn't know if I was running any faster.

The test came a few weeks later, in the Manchester 10k Run. I had completed it with my *BBC Breakfast* co-presenter Bill Turnbull the year before and finished in what seemed then to be a respectable time: 56.19 minutes. The reality was that I needed to lose several minutes off that time to have a chance of qualifying, so this was going to be a real test of my ability. It would put a marker down on whether I was going to be able to squeeze into the Great Britain triathlon team for my age group.

As luck would have it, Greg was starting the run that day, so it was fantastic to see him and have a last-minute pep talk before I set off. Claire, my coach, was running with me, which was very reassuring, because I had no idea at the time of how to pace myself over 10 kilometres. I bounced along to the music at the start, trying to warm up and prepare myself, and as Greg sounded the klaxon I set off as most people tend to do – far too fast. There was no way I would be able to keep up that kind of effort over the distance, so Claire told me to slow down as we jogged our way from the city centre towards Old Trafford.

The Great Manchester Run is a wonderful event, with an electrifying atmosphere and hundreds of supporters out on the streets shouting encouragement. Even so, it still felt incredibly hard work, especially on the way back.

I was just about on track for a good time, with about one kilometre to go, when Claire told me to try a bit harder. Even thinking about it now makes me feel nauseous. I forced myself to run as hard as I could, getting to the line absolutely spent – gasping for air and feeling considerably worse than after finishing the year before. Once I could breathe properly again, I was desperate for the result. Seven months into my training, and a year on from my last 10k run, had all that hard work made a difference? What would I do if it had made little or no difference?

We waited for the results text message – and hooray! It had! I might have been feeling terrible, but I had finished in 51.42. A fat four and a half minutes quicker than the year before. Finally, my running was heading in the right direction. So how would that affect my triathlon times?

The next test was the Chirk triathlon in April 2015, run by Wrexham Tri Club, which is Chester Tri Club's nearest neighbour. It is a popular event and entries for the race sell out within minutes of going online.

Among members of Chester Tri Club, Chirk is the first real test of the triathlon season, so the atmosphere tends to be very focused and intense. Everyone is keen to post a fast time to show how hard they have been training over the winter. I was astonished to see how many athletes from Chester Tri were there, and it was great to be one of them – but their presence really added to the pressure.

The 400-metre swim was in an indoor pool. Unlike the race in Machynlleth, though, it wasn't a system of first come, first served. Your time in the pool was allocated according to your predicted swim time, so the slower swimmers went in first. This meant I had to wait a while before I jumped in to start my race. I didn't enjoy the swim, feeling too hot, and distracted by the other swimmers alongside me, behind me or in front of me. They all looked so much faster than I was. In my haste, I took more than a few gulps of water, which had me spluttering, and I also managed to get water in one side of my goggles. I swam on, with one eye closed, determined not to let that slow me down, and in fact it didn't seem to be too much of a problem. Until, that is, I got out of the pool and opened both eyes again, and realised that the contact lens had fallen out of my left eye. There was nothing I could do about it. I didn't have a spare one in transition; it had never occurred to me I would need one. With my vision seriously impaired, I had only two options: to continue with the race, seeing properly through only one eye, or to stop altogether. I realised that I wasn't going to get into the Great Britain triathlon team if I stopped for something so simple as a lost lens.

I could see clearly on my left only as far as my elbow, which made the customary challenges of finding everything in transition extremely difficult. Despite this, I scrabbled everything together and hopped on my bike to head out on the cycle route. A race official shouted at me. What had I done? This time, in the panic of not being able to see properly, I had managed to get on my bike before the mount line. I had to get off, turn around and start again.

David and the girls were there at the start of the cycle route to cheer me on, and witnessed my confusion. 'I have lost a contact lens!' I shouted out, to let them know what was going on.

Knowing how short-sighted I am, and that I would be finding the race tricky, they decided to chase me down on the cycle route so that they could pass me another lens.

What I know now, but didn't know then, was that handing me a spare was strictly not allowed under British Triathlon Rules and could have meant instant disqualification.

The rules are clear-cut: 'Compete without receiving assistance other than from event personnel and officials.' Unaware of this at the time, I was happy to see them by the side of the road, holding out a case, so I stopped. With my hands shaking from the adrenaline and the cold, I opened it – only to find it was empty.

I had wasted precious seconds messing about, and then had to cycle on without it.

On the straight bits of road, I felt OK, but cornering at speed on my bike, able to see clearly through only one eye, was alarming. I couldn't judge distances, and discovered that I could negotiate the corners safely only by closing my affected eye and holding on for dear life.

Despite the optical challenges, I was surprised to enjoy the bike ride into the Welsh hills, with the wind blowing in my face, and took delight in successfully holding my line on a sharp left-hand turn over a bridge to hear the river gushing beneath it. With all the distractions, the turnaround point at just over 10 kilometres seemed to arrive quickly, and I headed back to transition feeling confident and fast.

I was relieved to make it back in one piece, and knew that at the speed I run, seeing with one eye only wasn't going to be problematic. (This could be the only time I have looked forward to the run on a triathlon.)

What I remember most about the route, apart from one tough hill that came right at the start and which was repeated at the end, was all the other Chester Tri Club members shouting encouragement as they passed me. That made it feel like a great race and a great day out.

So how had I done? Was I making progress towards the Great Britain triathlon team?

The 400-metre swim was respectably under seven minutes (6.58). I finished the half-sighted 23-kilometre bike ride in 48.15 minutes, and the 5-kilometre run in a pleasing 25.37 minutes, edging closer to my target of under 25 minutes. I was ninth in my age group, in a very competitive race, so I had done well – but there was definitely work to do, particularly because all the distances in my qualifying races would be doubled.

Most importantly of all, I had come away having learned three extremely important lessons.

The first was to prepare properly. In the future, I would have everything I needed to race with me in transition, and that meant *everything*. From that race on, I have always made sure I have a spare contact lens Sellotaped to my bike frame, just in case. In fact, I pretty much have a spare everything: googles, tri belt, shoes, gels.

Secondly, when things go wrong, get on with it. Even if it feels challenging at the time, knuckle down and work around it. You can still carry on and finish a race.

Thirdly, read the rules carefully – and obey them! If you don't know what they are, you are likely to break them, and therefore very likely to get yourself disqualified. All that hard work and effort will count for nothing.

CHAPTER 12

THE THRILL OF THE RACE

'I had given it my all and looked like a wreck when I staggered out of the river, dripping with water and struggling to catch my breath.'

Swimming has always been the discipline I am best at in triathlon, but every second counts, so it had to improve.

My swim in the pool at Chirk had gone well, and I had been second in my age group, but I didn't know if my speed was improving in open water.

I spent numerous early summer evenings braving the swimming lakes in Cheshire, but nothing beats race conditions and I soon found an opportunity to see if I was getting quicker. I had entered the Dee Mile, which is not a race of a mile, as the name suggests, but a slightly longer 2-kilometre race downstream in the River Dee, ending up in Chester.

It is a very popular race, with a couple of hundred people taking part every year. It also has a competitive atmosphere, especially among the Chester Tri Club because it is their local race and they all want to beat each other. After the race briefing, the competitors walked across the Meadows to the riverbank.

I am not sure why, but I felt unorganised and nervous at the start. I cheered up, though, when I saw we were divided into two different waves, with the faster swimmers going off first. The first section was mainly made up of men and I was happy to be assigned to the second wave; I wasn't in the mood to get mixed up in the macho mêlée.

It was a beautiful warm summer's evening, and fun to be watching and offering encouragement from the sidelines as the first wave started their journey downstream. Five minutes or so after they departed, we were beckoned into the water. Once my toes were in, I felt immediately much calmer, thinking that it might possibly be a good night for a swim.

Compared to both the previous times I had raced in the river – terrified in the triathlon, then frozen during the 5-kilometre swim – this race was a joy. From the start, I had clear, open water in front of me, and no one bashing me from the side. I was no longer afraid of the lack of visibility. I felt happy and able to relax and let the current help me along.

To my surprise, I was swimming so efficiently that by about halfway through I started catching up with the swimmers in front of me and even overtaking some of them, which made me more determined to try even harder and speed up towards the finish.

I had given it my all and looked like a wreck as I staggered out of the river, dripping with water and struggling to catch my breath. Seeing how many people from the first wave I had managed to overtake, I knew the effort had been worth it.

All those months in the pool, with endless lengths and boring training drills, had paid off.

That beautiful summer night, I had swum the two kilometres in 29 minutes and 38 seconds. Most excitingly, I had come 14th out of 111 women in the race. I could celebrate: my swimming was indeed getting faster, exactly what I needed.

I was as ready as I could be to put all the disciplines to the test.

CHAPTER 13

DOUBLING THE DISTANCE

'Come on! Stop being so silly, this is all ridiculous. Just stop and pack it in.'

There was so much riding on that first qualifier.

I had worked so hard to get myself fit enough to be there and, in the weeks before, I had really begun to feel the pressure.

I knew I had trained as hard and as often as I possibly could, squeezing it in around work and home, but I felt like all the effort just wasn't going to be enough. A friend of mine told me I looked exhausted, and suggested I take some time off before the race to recharge my batteries. I listened to his advice, and took a day off work in the week of the race, hoping that one less alarm call at 3.40 a.m. might make the difference to my legs.

Race-day was going to be a day of intimidating firsts.

For a start, it was the first time I had ever raced Standard or Olympic distance, so there was no guarantee I could even complete the course.

It was also the first time I had ever raced in a qualifier. Until that point, I competed in triathlons that were fun races with nothing more at stake than finishing and trying to beat my own times. In stark contrast, at the Deva Triathlon, triathletes from all over the UK would be there, honed and ready to fight for their right to wear a Great Britain triathlon team suit.

It would have been ultra-competitive had it just been a World Championship qualifier, but that year the race was a 'double' qualifier. There were places for both the World Championships and the European Championships up for grabs, which meant that even more top athletes would be out on the course, adding even more pressure. What's more, it was also the Triathlon England Standard Distance National Championships, so everyone who was anyone in the GB triathlon age-group world would be there.

I had no choice, though. This was the moment I had chosen. So, ready or not, I had to do my best. Otherwise, all those months of training would come to nothing.

I knew that being organised on the day was going to make a big difference to the way I felt going into the race.

To try and remove as many worries and niggles as I possibly could, I registered and collected my race pack the night before. I almost wished I hadn't. The atmosphere in the registration hall in Chester was intense: there were dozens of lean and keen triathletes of all ages, looking fit, strong and confident, and chatting about race strategy as they carb-loaded with steaming plates of pasta. Seeing them did nothing to calm my nerves.

Being on home turf, I already knew the course well, but I listened carefully as the organisers went through a detailed race briefing and described things to watch out for on the route.

The 1,500-metre swim was in my favourite river, the Dee. It streams right past my house, and this is where I had lost my fear of deep and murky water. Most of the race would be upstream, starting from the jetty by the ornate octagonal cast-iron bandstand on The Groves. It then went under the Iron Bridge, where I had nearly passed out after the big river swim, and all the way up to the King's School Rowing Club, around a buoy and back down to the Boathouse Inn. Finally, there was a steep run up to transition in wonderful Victorian Grosvenor Park.

The cycle leg was a huge scenic loop that headed out beneath the historic city's rose-coloured walls, over the sandstone Old Dee Bridge, then into the countryside through Rossett and into Wales, back over the Dee again and along the river, finally arriving in the park for transition. I knew the cycle route well, having ridden it many times before. Apart from one hill it should, I thought, be very fast, especially on a downhill section of dual carriageway.

The run was on the Chester Meadows, with a stunning view of the houses overlooking the river. It was where I had done my first ever triathlon, the Deva Divas, but this time it was three laps of the route and double the distance – 10 kilometres instead of five kilometres.

I was determined to be completely organised. I laid out all my kit at home in the exact order I would need things, looking carefully at where I was going to put everything in transition and working out what would be the easiest – and, of course, the quickest – way of doing things.

My nerves were already tickling at my insides, but I calmed down a bit when our friends from London, Ian Blandford and Jay Hunt, arrived. They had made a huge effort to get there to support me, and it was meant to be a surprise, but one of the children let the cat out of the bag. I did a rubbish job of pretending I didn't know they were coming because I was so excited.

I have learned that sometimes the best thing for my pre-race nerves is to be on my own. So, I woke early, had the regulatory porridge for breakfast, stuffed all my kit into a rucksack and cycled my way to the start. As I was heading into Chester, I could hear the loudspeaker echoing across the water, starting the earlier waves of swimmers. I was astonished to catch a glimpse of the leaders of the male cyclists thunder across the Old Dee Bridge, heads down and legs pumping, going past me in the opposite direction at what seemed to me to be superhuman speed. It was incredibly intimidating, and left my nerves jangling. A voice in my head said *Turn back now.* It was only the shame of giving up before I had even started that made me carry on.

Transition was incredibly busy.

It felt like the first day at a new school. Everyone seemed to know each other and exactly what they were doing, except for me. I couldn't even find where to put my bike. I managed to stay relatively calm, though, and set everything up just as I had practised. I even managed to remember Claire's instruction to do a dummy run of the entrances and exits so that when I came out discombobulated from the swim I would know which lane of cycles to turn into and how far I would have to run to my bike.

I tried not to be distracted by the added pressure of being filmed by both the BBC and Channel 4. *Breakfast* had sent a camera crew, just in case I qualified, and the Channel 4 camera crew were filming that day for a programme about GB age-groupers.

There was time for a quick goodbye to David and the girls, and Jay and Ian. Just before I left, Jay gave me the most fantastic – and opportune – piece of advice. She looked at me very seriously and said, 'Remember how much you have put into this. Remember how much we all support you. And, most importantly, remember this: Don't fuck it up!'

Some people might not take that kind of advice very well. For me, though, it was brilliant: all the worries in the world disappeared and nothing else mattered. All I needed to do was not mess up! That, I could handle.

Claire, my coach, was also racing that day, and even though she was in a different age group, we were in the same swimming wave. It meant we could start next to each other in the water – and, if all went well, I could try to stick beside or behind her, and draft off her feet or hips, which is allowed in the swim. Swimming close behind another swimmer means you are carried along in their slipstream.

We were part of the first group to jump into the deep dark water, and I set off with a cheery wave, making my way to the far side where we thought the current flowing downstream wouldn't be so fast. Claire was very reassuring, treading water beside me and telling me that the hard work was done now. All I had to do was race hard and try and enjoy it. We jostled for position, trying to find a space among the bobbing red hats, and I waited with my heart racing for the starting gun.

The gun went off, and the churning mass of swimmers turned the water white. It was like being inside a washing machine, tumbled by other swimmers' arms, hands, elbows and feet as we all reached forward, pushing and pulling in the struggle to get ahead. I held my nerve, and focused on trying to stay with Claire. I caught a glimpse of what I thought were her feet kicking ahead of me, and concentrated on them, following as closely as I could. After a couple of hundred metres, we reached the Iron Bridge, the field started to spread out, and we found ourselves swimming in calm water, clear of other athletes.

I reached that amazing moment, which is one of the reasons that I train in the first place: the pre-race nerves vanish as if they had never existed and I start loving the feeling of swimming fast. I trusted that Claire would know exactly where she was going, so I didn't worry about looking up and trying to spot the buoys ahead. I just swam as quickly as possible, almost tickling her feet to keep up with her.

Unlike a 750-metre swim, 1,500 metres seems to give me time to think, sometimes just a little too much – and just before the last turn, I began to wonder if in fact I was swimming behind Claire at all. I started to doubt that we were going in the right direction, and decided to take a different route towards the exit. When I am racing in open water, I find it very difficult to tell where other people are, even if they are right beside me. Just before I got out, and to my shame, I pushed down hard with my right hand right on to the back of another swimmer. I had no idea she was there and felt terrible as we were both hauled to our feet on to the platform. Such collisions are part of the sport and all triathletes have accidentally given or received the occasional knock, but I still felt bad about it.

I was gasping for breath as I tore off my hat and goggles and tried to force my legs to run up the hill to transition. I knew I had tried hard, but it had felt really tough, and I was sure I hadn't been very fast. David was there, though, and shouted, 'Great swim, 23 minutes'. Wow! I was made up: a whole two minutes faster than I had hoped for. It had been a cracking swim, and I had come out of the water fourth out of 32 women in my age group.

The first transition, or T1, went well and I managed to rip off my wetsuit and get on my bike safely and quickly. I think both of the camera crews missed me because neither expected me to be so quick.

When I started the bike leg, I was in a great position and well ahead of most of the field. Even though my hands and feet were numb from the cold water, the first 25 kilometres of the cycle route were fantastic. I felt like I was flying, and I was loving every second. I even raced easily up the hardest hill, and hit a bone-shaking 35 miles per hour on a long downhill stretch of dual carriageway with the wind whistling loudly in my ears.

But my inexperience racing the longer distance became painfully obvious when we turned back towards Chester. I just didn't have the energy in my legs to maintain the speed, and then came the devastating moment when my fellow age-groupers started to catch me up.

I clearly remember Morag McDowall, who is now a friend, saying 'Nice bike' as she flew past me. I kept pushing but felt increasingly demoralised to be overtaken by what seemed to be a never-ending stream of women, all looking incredibly powerful and fast. What made it worse was that I could identify the women in my age group by the huge capital 'I' written on their leg next to their number. The 'I' meant they were part of the 45–50-year-old age group and the women I was trying to beat. Try as I might, I just didn't have the strength to keep up.

By the time I got back to transition, ready to get off my bike, my legs were spent.

David ran up beside me and warned me to take care: lots of people were falling off at the dismount line. I slowed down and dismounted carefully, but I could hardly stand, let alone run, and I hobbled as I pushed my bike back to the rack and put my running shoes on. I grabbed an energy gel, in the hope that would restore me, and set off down the hill towards the Meadows. After only 200 metres, I realised my shoes were annoying me, and I looked down to see one of my laces had come undone. I had to fix it, so I bent down to do it up, losing about 30 valuable seconds.

As I had that little breather, the voice in my head said, 'Come on! Stop being so silly, this is all ridiculous. Just stop and pack it in. You can hardly run five kilometres. How are you going to run 10?'

But I knew that everyone was waiting for me on the bridge and remembered Jay's advice. 'Don't fuck it up.' Right then, in my head that meant, 'Don't give up.'

The fantastic thing about the Deva course was that, because it was three laps, my family and friends could shout encouragement at me in at least six different places. Every time I wanted to walk or give up altogether, they would appear again, pushing me onwards.

Everything hurt: my lungs hurt, my legs hurt, my feet hurt, even my wrists and eyelids hurt. If that were not bad enough, I was feeling dispirited by continually being overtaken. I eventually realised the only way I was going to get through the 10 kilometres was by sticking with someone else.

When I had stopped to tie my shoelace, an older gentleman passed me. Over and over again on the course we kept passing each other, and started chatting and encouraging each other along the way. When he passed me for about the fifth time, on the final lap, I thought, *Right, that is it, I am going to stay with him to the finish line – and if he makes it, so will I.*

It was like being pulled along on a lifeline. As soon as I focused on following in his footsteps, I stopped thinking about the pain and became mesmerised by his feet pounding along the tarmac. On and on we went until we hit the final turn. Seeing the finish line ahead, I managed one last huge effort: picking up my feet, I sprinted as best as I possibly could across the line, my arms aloft. I felt incredibly proud, exhilarated – and absolutely spent.

As I plonked my head down between my hands on one of the barriers to try and get my breath back, I was overcome. I had given it my absolute best. I hadn't let those doubting demons in my head get the better of me and make me stop, turn back or walk. I had kept on going despite being constantly overtaken. And, most importantly of all, I hadn't fucked it up!

Fittingly, Nadia Dahabiyeh – the *BBC Breakfast* producer who had prompted me to take up the triathlon in the first place by creating that bike race in the Velodrome – was the first person to rush up and congratulate me. She was closely followed by Mia, Scarlett and the rest of my enthusiastic supporters, who nearly suffocated me with hugs. I had finished the run in 52 minutes, 42 seconds, only one minute slower than my fastest ever 10k.

But had I managed to qualify?

When I picked up my finishing time with my medal, it showed that I completed the course in 2 hours, 38 minutes and 3 seconds.

I had been fast in the swim, fourth in my age group, but after that I had slipped right down the leader board to 20th out of 32. It was clear I wasn't going to have an automatic qualifying place – that required placing in the top four – but all was not lost. I might just have a qualifying time. If I did, that would make me eligible for a roll-down place.

My finishing time would have to be within 115 per cent of the woman who had won my age group: Sheila Jansen, who had finished in 2 hours, 20 minutes, 11 seconds. Each of her other split times was staggeringly impressive: a mere 20 minutes, 47 seconds on the swim; just over 1 hour, 13 minutes on the bike, a full five minutes ahead of me; and then, to finish, a super-speedy 43 minutes on her run. What a legend! The only place that I had been quicker than her was in T1, where I managed to get in and out two seconds faster than she did – something of a miracle.

We tried to do the maths and work out how close I was to Sheila's winning time. We reckoned that I might have been just fast enough to get within that crucial 115 per cent for a qualifying time. But there was an added complication. I had taken those extra 30 seconds or so tying up my lace, so there were at least two other athletes who had been a few seconds faster, meaning they were now ahead of me in the roll-down places. Even though I would most likely have a qualifying time, I was some way off having a guaranteed place.

Yet I didn't care about times and qualifying. I felt elated: it had been a hard race, and I felt a huge sense of achievement. I had successfully completed the distance and, what's more, I had enjoyed it. More than anything, I had loved beating myself, not listening to the part of me that says, *You can't do this, it is too hard, stop, turn back, go home.* My body was aching, but I was on an irrepressible high.

I knew I had tried my best on the day, so I wasn't disappointed or annoyed with myself about my performance, but I did have to accept the fact that despite those months of training, the dedication, the effort and the hard work, and the impact on my family, I just wasn't good enough. So what was I going to do?

I could have rested on my laurels and waited to see what happened with roll-down, but the wait would have been months. For a real sense of achievement and pride, I knew I would have to try again.

Just a couple of hours after I finished the race, Claire confirmed what I had already guessed: I hadn't automatically qualified. If I wanted a guaranteed chance of getting to the World Championships, I was going to have to race again – and race faster.

There was only one chance left, and that was in a mere six days' time: the alarmingly named Dambuster Triathlon in Rutland Water. I had less than a week to recover, and would have to be ready to compete all over again.

In my mind, I had no choice at all.

I was within touching distance of that crazy goal, the GB Team strip. Not only was I determined to get into the team, I wanted to do it with my head held high thanks to an automatic qualification place. I didn't want to be in the awkward position of waiting to see who dropped out or didn't want their slot.

So that was how it had to be: from never having completed one Olympic distance race, I would now be attempting two races within one week.

At least I knew I could go the distance.

CHAPTER 14

CONQUERING THE DEMONS

'Don't be ridiculous! You want to be in the Great Britain triathlon team. You can't possibly get off your bike and walk.'

Give it up now. It's agony. Stop running, you idiot. You are so stupid. What on earth do you think you are doing? You are never going to get into the Great Britain triathlon team. What a ridiculous idea! You can't do this. You can't run one kilometre, so why are you trying to run 10? It is impossible. Get over yourself. Walk now, give up and go back to the start.

I was just one kilometre into the 10-kilometre run at the Dambuster Triathlon, my last opportunity to get into the Great Britain Age-Group Team, and I felt like I was drowning in a tsunami of negative thoughts, smashing into each other in my brain, their noise and distraction overwhelming me. And I believed each of them. What was I doing and why was I doing it? At that moment, I had no answer and no defence. I had no choice. I decided I was going to stop, turn around and walk back to the start.

But as my feet slowed down, visions of my family flashed before my eyes. I could imagine the disappointment on their faces when they realised that I had given up. All along, they had been an integral part of the mad adventure. They had gone out of their way to support me in everything I had done. Cycling alongside me while I ran, rowing down the river in Chester while I swam, and coming to every single race to cheer me on. They had been unflinchingly loyal, supportive and encouraging in my every endeavour.

This time, I had really pushed it. I had dragged them halfway across the country on a horrible long and wet Friday night drive. Then woken them up at 4 a.m. on a Saturday morning, to make them stand at dawn by a lake in the drizzle while I was fiddling about with my bike, being annoying, fidgety and nervous. And I knew that right then, while I was vacillating and about to pack it all in, they would be waiting anxiously, watching out for me, hoping beyond hope that I would be OK and that, having tried my best, I had got into the team.

I have never felt such a powerful wave of determination driving me forward. There was no way I could let them down now. They thought I could finish the race, so I would have to finish the race. However much it hurt, I was going to keep on running and ignore those persistent demons in my head. I had a sudden moment of clarity. If I stopped, I would be letting myself down and my family down too, and there would be no way back from that: they would never forget and I, in turn, would never forgive myself.

The six days between the Deva Triathlon and the Dambuster Triathlon had gone in a flash.

I had tried to concentrate on recovering from the exertion at the same time as getting up early to present *Breakfast*. Mentally, I felt elated; physically, I was a wreck, with aching heavy legs, nausea and no appetite. Two days after the race, I looked as if I had lost about half a stone. Something should have been telling me that I had failed to get my nutrition right, and was probably a bit dehydrated too, but it didn't.

Logistics around Dambuster were obviously going to be much more stressful than competing at home. I also didn't have a clue about what the course was like, so I looked up the description on the Internet. What I saw filled me with dread.

First, it wasn't a deep-water start, which I was now confident I could manage, but a beach start. Everyone had to line up near the water's edge and then, when the klaxon blasted, dash hell for leather into the lake, running as far as they could before being tripped up by the deeper water. If you knew what you were doing, and timed it right, you would then dive in and effortlessly start to swim. To me, it looked chaotic and dangerous.

The bike ride was a 42-kilometre loop around Rutland Water. The website described it as follows: 'Good testing course and well suited to strong bikers. Best described as undulating, it's sure to sort out the standings. The Rutland Ripple is not the only test of endurance on the course which offers little in the way of flat.'

Goodness me! 'Strong bikers', 'little in the way of flat', and what on earth was the Rutland Ripple? If I had struggled around the much less challenging course in Chester the week before, how was I going to cope with that? The only positive thing I could read on the website was that there was a good road surface. Thank goodness!

The description of the run wasn't much more encouraging. The 10-kilometre course would navigate around the side of the lake and over the dam after which the triathlon was named. The most worrying part was the warning on the website: 'Don't be deceived by the flatness of the run section . . . The fact that you can see the competition for much of the run means this is a psychologically challenging course.'

A psychologically challenging course? I always find the run the most mentally challenging part of a race anyway, so was this going to be even harder than normal?

Despite my misgivings, I knew that there was no alternative. If I wanted any chance of qualifying for the Great Britain Age-Group Team, I was going to have to give it a go. That was why we had ended up by the lake at dawn.

After the girls finished school on Friday night, we packed the car to the gunnels with all my tri gear, and managed to squeeze Mia, Scarlett, Waffle the Labrador and my bike in the back. We arrived at the hotel in Corby at about ten o'clock at night – way too late for my liking. It was going to be an incredibly quick turnaround. To be at transition in time to register and pick up my race pack, we had to be in the car again by 4 a.m. The girls were not impressed!

In the early hours, I put on my tri suit and realised that I had forgotten my sports bra.

You might not think that sounds like a problem, but it completely threw me. What was I going to do? I really didn't want to run or bike without one; I would be both incredibly self-conscious and uncomfortable. Thankfully, I had packed two tri suits, so my only alternative was to wear them both, one on top of the other. That might make me feel better! I squeezed myself into them and even though it was a tight fit, I did feel much better; there was no danger of anything bouncing around!

When we arrived at Rutland Water, a grey mist was clinging to the black lake. In the dark I joined a line of triathletes pushing their bikes purposefully over the grass towards the registration tent. Once again it felt like everyone knew each other except for me, and they looked intimidatingly fit and focused.

The race briefing, issued shortly after dawn, was both formidable and unnerving.

This time, it was for all the competitors, huddled together shivering by the lakeside café, and the atmosphere was much more competitive than at the previous week's Deva Triathlon. It was made clear that any infringement of the rules would be taken extremely seriously.

Over the loudspeaker, we were given a stark reminder of the things we must not do. 'Any use of profanity or aggression towards any other parties will result in an immediate Disqualification from the event and a ban from all future events hosted by both the venue and the promoters. If you are spotted littering on the bike or other areas of the run this is an instant Disqualification – you've been warned.'

We were also reminded that the bike section was strictly a non-drafting race. Taking advantage of anyone's slipstream was illegal. To enforce this, they had eight referees on motorbikes, who were going to be out on the course all day. It was going to be quite a challenge.

The first wave of competitors to set off was the 17–35 male age-groupers. There were 179 of them. Dressed in their slick black wetsuits, they looked like seals racing for the ocean, splashing into the water, and bouncing through it to try to get as deep as they could before diving in to swim. Watching them, I tried to work out if it was faster to run further in the shallow water on the right-hand side, or whether I should just take my chances and go for it in the middle. Having never done a beach start before, I was unable to decide.

I was in the last wave, and there were 90 of us in the 45–75 age group. I knew I had to steel myself and get out at the front if I was going to take advantage of my swimming ability. As always, I was shivering and shaking with nerves, and my feet were already feeling cold as I stood on the water's edge. But I was ready, and as the whistle went, I sprinted as fast as I could into the shallows, jumping over the water, and when it got too deep to run, diving in to start swimming.

The water was heavenly: clear and calm. After the first 100 metres, I could see only one woman steaming away ahead of me and another swimming alongside me. By the first buoy, the triathlete on my left slipped ahead of me and I settled in to swim behind her, making sure to draft behind her, following the bubbles made by her feet. Even though I was swimming as fast as I could, I felt incredibly calm as I gazed down into the beautiful, deep blue water. I felt utterly in my element and the distance markers just kept coming with what seemed not much effort at all. At the final turn, back towards the jetty, I decided I could put in some more effort, and overtook the woman who I had been with most of the way, taking what I thought was a more direct line towards the exit.

I was ecstatic to come out of the water third. It was a huge boost to my confidence as I raced to my bike. The double tri suit solution worked a treat, and had the added advantage of making me feel a little warmer as I set off over the hills. The legendary Rutland Ripple, which turned out to be a set of three undulating hills one after the other, was not the daunting challenge I had expected but turned out to be great fun. I found that if I was brave enough, and held on tight to my shaking bike as I cycled down one side of the hills at maximum speed, I picked up a momentum that would carry me a long way up the other side to do it all over again. It was faster than I have ever ridden before, and the speed was exhilarating.

After the Ripple, things began to feel a bit tougher. Ahead of me, on a steep hill, I could see both men and women getting off their bikes and starting to push them up the sharp incline. My legs were burning with the effort and it was incredibly tempting to do the same, but a voice in my head said, 'Don't be ridiculous! You want to be in the Great Britain triathlon team. You can't possibly get off your bike and walk. Get out of your saddle, stand on your pedals, and get a move on!'

I did.

I flew round the rest of the course and, for the first time in my triathlon career, found myself overtaking people on the way. It was going brilliantly until the last kilometre, when I had to brake hard as a pedestrian stepped out to cross the road in front of me. To my shame, I shouted just as a moto-referee passed beside me. The strict race briefing replayed in my mind, and I was mortified. Would I be disqualified? I just hoped the referee hadn't heard me.

I took the last descent down to the lake at top speed and dashed into transition and out in record time, only to be shouted at by race officials. I had done it again: I was so paranoid about taking my helmet off too soon, and getting disqualified for taking it off before I racked my bike, that I had entirely forgotten it was still on my head, and I was running out with it firmly clasped under my chin. I had to turn round and run all the way back to my bike to leave it there, losing precious seconds.

Up until that point, everything had gone as well as I could possibly have hoped. So it was a shock when I smashed into that brick wall of self-doubt a mere one kilometre into the run. The remaining nine kilometres stretched before me like an impassable mountain. The race organisers were right about the psychologically challenging course. Runners streamed towards me from across the dam, well on their way to finishing their race and I was only heading out.

I had won the first skirmish in the battle against those overwhelming negative thoughts, but there was still a long way to get back to my family, so I had to come up with another way to distract myself.

I started counting my steps, one to a hundred, over and over, again and again. Very slowly the metres became kilometres, and they all added up. The race is now a blur, but I vaguely remember reaching the turnaround and passing Rutland's famous landmark, Normanton Church, to see the incongruous sight of wedding guests all dressed immaculately in suits and dresses, wandering over to watch us sweating in our tri suits. I kept pushing forward, and every time a runner passed me – and many did – I would put in an extra burst of speed, trying as best I could to keep up with their footsteps and using their energy to help carry me on.

On the last bend I saw the sailing boats lined up against one another, masts flapping in the breeze, and knew that the end was finally in sight. I was so excited, I summoned a last burst of energy and threw my hands up in the air as I crossed the finish line. It had been a monumental effort, a battle over self-doubt, and I was overwhelmed and close to tears as I collapsed into the arms of my patient, waiting family.

Qualification for the Great Britain triathlon team was the last thing on my mind. The most important thing was that I had managed to beat my own negative thoughts.

After a short recovery, which included downing a pint of non-alcoholic beer being handed out at the finish, I went to find my results. How had I done?

The swim had gone well: I finished the 1,500 metres in 25 minutes, 22 seconds. It was slower than my swim at the Deva Triathlon, where the current had been with me, but I had still emerged from the water at the top of my age group. At 1 hour, 27 minutes, the bike was slower too, but it had been a longer course, with those challenging hills, and looking at the timings revealed that most people had found it difficult. The run had felt like agony, but I had managed it in 53.11, only 30 seconds more than the 10 kilometres the week before, which was a remarkable achievement given how overwhelmed I had felt. Overall, the race had taken me 2 hours, 48 minutes, 55 seconds. A whopping 11 minutes over my time for the previous Qualifier. But did that matter? This was a different course, so how had everyone else done?

Their results, as well as mine, would be the key to my future in the Great Britain triathlon team.

I waited anxiously in the queue for the little white slip of paper with my race statistics. When I could decipher it, the results revealed some exciting news. I had moved up 13 places in the rankings, coming seventh in my age group. I wasn't in the top four in my age group, so I didn't have an automatic place in the team, but I could at least be in with a chance.

On the way home, I would have to look at the fine print of the British Triathlon Federation Rules. I knew getting a qualifying place wasn't going to be straightforward.

According to those BTF rules, my finish time needed to be within 115 per cent of the winner of my age group on the day. That was Anita Howe, who I had also raced against in Chester. She had finished Dambuster in a very impressive 2 hours, 27 minutes, 16 seconds – more than 21 minutes ahead of me. David and I tried to do the maths, and reckoned that I might possibly be within a few seconds of having a good enough time, but we couldn't be entirely sure. We would have to wait for the BTF website to confirm it.

Thank goodness I hadn't given in and got off my bike and walked up those hills, but leaving my helmet on and having to run back to put it on the bike could possibly be the mistake that cost me a place.

I would also have to wait and see how many of the six people who had beaten me had registered their interest in a place in the Great Britain Age-Group Team. There were four qualifying places available on the day. I was pretty sure that Anita had a guaranteed place at the Triathlon World Championships in Chicago because of her time at the Deva Triathlon, so she didn't need one of them. That meant there were possibly five of us going for the four remaining places. But who else had registered? I didn't know.

As we drove home, I felt physically broken. That day, I had raced as hard as I possibly could have. There was nothing more that I could have done. Now, all I could do was wait, and the wait would be agonising.

Almost hourly for the next few days I checked the BTF website. I even phoned them up, but there was nothing they could tell me until all the results had been verified. Finally, I got a very short text from Claire, my coach.

'You've done it!'

Had I? Really?

I wouldn't believe it until I saw it with my own eyes, and when I looked at the website for the 100th time, there, beside my name in black and white was a new mark: Q2.

'Q' for qualified. Oh yes! I really had done it; I was now in the Great Britain triathlon team! And '2' meant that I had qualified in second place. What a marvel! That was what I had worked for. I was incredibly proud.

All those months juggling work with hard training, dragging myself out on cold wet runs, hauling myself up and down the swimming pool, and over hills on my bike – every single minute of effort had added up together to make a place in the team possible.

What had started out as a hugely ambitious and ridiculous dream was now a reality. At the start it seemed absurd and impossible, but I had dared to try and had pulled it off. I was going to represent my country in sport on an international stage.

What a fabulous adventure it had been, and it wasn't over yet. I was going to represent Great Britain in the World Triathlon Championships in Chicago.

CHAPTER 15

A TRIATHLETE'S KIT

'Vaseline and talcum powder are a triathlete's best friends.'

I wasn't ready for the inundation of information after I qualified.

In all those hard months of training and racing, I had never dared to dream that I would actually qualify for the team, so I was unprepared for the influx of emails from both the International Triathlon Union and the British Triathlon Federation about the World Championships.

Over the next few weeks I was slightly flustered about the amount of things I had to organise. First came a message of congratulations from the Team Manager, along with a brilliant piece of advice: 'Good luck with your final preparations, do not fret over matters you can't control, concentrate on what you can control and influence.'

That was followed by a series of questions to answer and forms to fill out. How was I going to get my bike to America? What kind of visa did I need? Did I need race insurance? Did I want to take part in the Parade of Nations? It was never-ending.

The most exciting email of all told me how to buy my team kit. I duly went on the website and ordered myself a tri suit, swimming hat, T-shirt and top.

The moment my GB Team tri suit arrived has to be one of my most exciting and proud moments ever. It was a skimpy Lycra number in red, white and blue, and written in giant capitals across my chest were the magic words MINCHIN GBR. Those months of hard work paid off, and I was worthy of wearing it – I could barely believe it.

My GB tri suit was the most fabulous addition to my ever-expanding triathlon kit. When I first started my triathlon journey, not only had I had no idea, I also had none of the gear. Over the years that had changed incrementally, and I have now collected a large amount of kit which I take to races, everything from the obvious bike, wetsuit, and cycle helmet, to the not so obvious spare contact lenses and lucky laces.

One of the most challenging things I find about competing is remembering to take everything I need on the day to make sure I can race as fast and efficiently as possible. To make it easier and avoid silly mistakes and forgetting things, I have written myself a list, which I go through a couple of days before I compete.

- Race pack and rules – the list starts with my race pack and a print out of the rules. I try and read the rules for each triathlon a few days before, and then again on the way there, as every race can be slightly different. Most importantly I check and double-check where and what time registration starts and what time it closes. There is nothing worse than turning up and missing registration or your race wave. It will depend on the race, but sometimes you are sent your numbers, race timing chip and swim hat in an envelope before the day of the race. If that is the case, I always check everything is in it, then put it back in the envelope and make sure I take it with me. I don't want to turn up without the right swimming hat, or without a timing chip – it would just be too stressful.

- High on the list is my Triathon England Membership Card and Race Licence. Each home nation – England, Wales and Scotland – has its own association and issues membership cards which serve as identification so you can pick up your race-pack and insurance for the day.

After those essentials, I then organise my packing into what I need for each discipline. For the swim leg, this is what I need:

- Tri suit – I wear my tri suit under my wetsuit. It is a hybrid of a swimming costume and a pair of cycling shorts, so it has padding on the bottom to make it more comfortable on the bike, and for modesty's sake, mine is less skimpy than a cozzie. I always tend to arrive already wearing my tri suit so I can't possibly leave it behind, and, having failed to take a sports bra to one of my World Championship Qualifiers, I also write that on the list and arrive wearing it!
- Wetsuit – if you are swimming in open water in the UK, because of the water temperature, most of the time it is compulsory to wear a wetsuit. Not only will it keep you warm but it also helps with buoyancy. No wetsuit can mean no race, so that has to be packed.
- Contact lenses – having had an epic failure and losing a contact lens in a race, I always pack extras, and have a spare lens taped to the frame of my bike in case one should ever fall out again.
- Swimming goggles – Because of my contact lenses, I can't swim without goggles and I am so paranoid about not having them with me, I always pack two pairs.
- Swim hat – most triathlons provide you with swim hats, as they are an easy way of identifying which wave of a race you are in, but I always take one just in case that doesn't happen. Some people like wearing two hats for warmth and comfort, but for me that would just be another thing to forget.

- Tri belt – I like wearing a belt around my waist with my number on it rather than pin numbers to my tri suit. Some races allow you to wear them over your tri suit and under your wetsuit, and if that is allowed I always do it, as it means in transition I don't have to remember to put on my number.
- Vaseline and talcum powder – Vaseline and talcum powder are a triathlete's best friends. If there is a bit of your tri suit or wetsuit that is going to rub, then if you rub Vaseline underneath it, you should be OK. Talcum powder is also brilliant, and I shake it into both my cycling and running shoes to help slip them on. It is especially helpful when your feet are wet.

For the cycle leg, this is what I need:

- Bike – my bike is obvious and essential, but if you are just starting out then at some triathlons you can hire a bike, like you can a swimming wetsuit. I always check the tyre pressure, and that the gears and brakes are working when I get there.
- Helmet – quite simply if you have no cycle helmet, you will not be allowed to race. Safety, as it should be, is paramount, and race officials will always check you are wearing your helmet and it is done up properly before they let you into transition.
- Sunglasses – I always take a pair of sunglasses for two reasons: sunshine in your eyes on the bike can be dangerous at high speeds, and they also stop me getting bugs in my eyes which I absolutely hate, so I wear sunglasses even on an overcast day.
- Water bottles – rehydrating is essential. I used to have just one bottle on the bike, but now have two – one with water and the other with a sugary drink to help with my energy levels. I also have a spare in transition in case of emergencies.
- Cycle shoes – after a debacle in transition where I failed to put on my new bike shoes (stupidly, I had failed to undo the fastenings!), I always make sure they are open under my bike

and ready to put on to avoid fiddling with the buckles. My shoes have special cleats that clip into the bike pedals to make this process quicker.

For the Run Leg, this is what I need:

- Running shoes – in a race I always have my running shoes laced with elastic laces, which you don't have to tie. They can save a huge amount of time, which is especially important in a short event, and means you just slip your shoes on and run.
- Extra energy gels – I try and be organised about nutrition, as I am not very good at eating either on the bike or on the run, so I have an energy gel open and ready in my bike shoes which I have when I finish the swim, another in my trainers which I have before the run, and one extra to stuff down my tri suit for when things are feeling really tough. If it is a long bike section, I will also break an energy bar into bite sizes, which I store in a bag on the crossbar, so I can eat tiny bits as I go along.

    I have learnt by trial and error to pack a few things for after the race. There is nothing worse than having to drive home in wet kit so it is essential to pack dry clothes and shoes, to change into and keep warm on the way home. I always take some extra food as well for when I finish, perhaps a banana or peanut butter sandwich, something that is easy to eat and won't make me feel sick.

There are also the added extras that I have discovered come in useful, and I'll pack if I have space:

- Bike pump – it is sensible to take one, and I mostly do, but if you have forgotten (which I have done), you don't need to worry, as you're surrounded by triathletes in transition and someone will have one you can borrow.
- Puncture repair kit, plus inner tubes that fit. That said, I don't tend to carry a repair kit on my bike during a short race. I

reckon that if I have a problem, the race will be over for me by the time I have fixed it, so I would either walk home, or hope the race officials would help me.

- Sun cream – you could be on a hot course for hours and get very burned. I have seriously underestimated the sun in Yorkshire, and as a result of getting very burnt, spent a whole summer with tri suit marks etched onto my back.
- Flip-flops – lots of competitors wear them in case they step on something sharp as they walk to the swim. If you leave them by the race start and don't make your way back to collect them most triathlons have a system where they are scooped up at the end of the race and given to charity.

There are also things which at the start of my triathlon adventure I thought I needed in a race, but actually don't at all!

- Socks – in a race, I never cycle or run in socks. Every second counts, and those extra seconds fiddling and putting them on could cost me a place. I might have to change my mind about that should I ever choose to race over a longer distance.
- Towel – again, there is no time for the luxury of drying. You need to get on your bike and start racing; it might feel chilly at first, but you will dry off and warm up quickly. There is a notable exception to my no towel rule. Depending on the race, you may or may not be allowed a towel in transition, but if you are, they are an excellent way of marking where your bike is, so read the rules and if towels are allowed, take a bright and garish one that you can spot easily. It will make your transition much less stressful.
- Gloves – once again, why waste the time trying to put them on?
- Extra layers – generally, these should be banned as time-wasters – unless you are cycling or running like I have in hail.
- Lipstick – never!

CHAPTER 16

IF YOU FALL, GET BACK UP AGAIN

'Even though I was injured, not for a second did I think about stopping.'

I expect any triathlon to be challenging, but some turn out to be far more so than I ever imagined.

Tri Liverpool in the summer of 2015 was one of those races. I had planned to do the Olympic distance (swim 1,500 metres, cycle 40 kilometres and run 10 kilometres) in the run-up to the World Championships in Chicago, and was really looking forward to it, especially as I had been asked to be an ambassador for the race. In the weeks before, though, I wasn't feeling great and had been inundated with work, so at the last minute I changed my mind and decided to do the shorter Sprint distance (swim 750 metres, cycle 20 kilometres, run five kilometres).

It was a horribly drizzly and chilly day as we lined up at the start on the Liverpool docks, just down from the famous Royal Liver building. The atmosphere was fantastic, though. I was a little nervous about the swim, which was to take place in the Kings Dock – quite different from the lakes and rivers where I usually swam.

As ever, I felt some initial pre-race anxiety, but it wasn't long before those nerves were being replaced with fleeting moments of adrenaline-fuelled excitement.

I was assigned to one of the last waves. It was a women's only wave and we all warmed up by jumping up and down and swinging our arms to loud thumping music. The first thing I noticed, as I jumped off the jetty into the water, was that it was salty. It had never occurred to me that we would be swimming in seawater, which immediately added to my buoyancy – and gave me a great confidence boost.

There weren't too many of us on the front at the start line, so instead of the washing-machine start I was now getting used to, with everyone vying for a competitive advantage, it was quite amicable and decorous. That didn't last long. As we headed under one of the road bridges, I ended up tangled with another woman, who kicked me in the face, probably unawares, and my goggles slipped off. Thank goodness they didn't completely fall off and just ended up round my neck. I didn't panic. I just stopped, gulped some air and then put the goggles on again. With them in place, I put my head down and went on swimming.

A few moments later, I had the most extraordinary experience. Powering through the water, I looked down and glimpsed what I thought were small blue fish, hanging weightless in the water beneath me. After a few minutes of happily swimming alongside them, I realised they were in fact jellyfish! Rather than being overcome by panic, I was overwhelmed by a sense of well-being and calm. Such was the serenity of the moment, I still recall it now whenever I am feeling nervous or stressed. The jellyfish were my swimming companions, and it was an honour to be swimming with them.

The feeling of calm wasn't to last, though. The race was about to get a lot more difficult.

I was one of the few women in my wave who had swum so fast that we caught up with the wave of swimmers ahead of us. As a result, it was a mighty scramble to get out of the water. I then had a long slippery run to transition in bare feet, and as I prepared to mount my bike the weather took a dramatic turn for the worse.

It began raining incredibly hard, and the temperature dropped considerably. Soon I was shivering with cold, almost uncontrollably, even though I was pedalling as fast as possible. At about 10 kilometres, around halfway through the cycle, I noticed that my left foot was numb. I initially presumed this was a result of the cold, but the numbness inched slowly up my leg, eventually reaching my hip. I tried as best I could to shake it off, jiggling about on my bike at the same time as trying to cycle fast.

As I came into transition I knew I had a problem. I took my foot out of the pedal, to get the blood flowing, but nothing made any difference. My foot remained numb.

How was I going to dismount? The only way I can get off my bike is by placing my left foot on the floor first – and that was the foot with the problem. Thinking fast, I remembered that on the way out I had seen metal barriers on each side of the track by the transition area. My best bet was to head towards the left-hand side, and make a grab for the barrier, hoping that I could put my foot down gently and stop safely. As I headed towards the barriers, I slowed down and hoped for the best.

Carefully braking and in great pain, I just managed to grab the rail in time. It certainly wasn't one of my smoothest stops. (So much for safe and elegant.)

My foot was completely numb. As I put it down, it seemed not to belong to me. I looked at it, willing it to hold my weight and let me stand, but nothing happened. My foot and my brain seemed utterly disconnected, and my foot crumpled beneath me. To save myself, I pitched forward over the handlebars, landing hard on the bike and the tarmac, and taking the impact on my hands, knees and elbow. Ouch!

I hadn't even finished the tumble before a race official kindly scooped me to my feet, saying: 'It's OK, your bike is fine!' That is the lunacy and brilliance of triathlon. My bike was fine, so my injuries were temporarily forgotten. I started running, pushing my bike into transition.

It was only when I put on my running shoes that I discovered blood pouring from one knee and an elbow. Not for a second did I think about stopping. Strangely, neither my bloodied knee nor my elbow seemed to hurt, and I could tell by the number of bikes not yet returned to transition that I was ahead of most of my age group. I was doing well, so I just carried on.

The conditions were bleak, rain pouring down hard with an icy chill. The Liverpool crowd was amazing, shouting encouragement from under their umbrellas. Still struggling with a numb foot, I wasn't going particularly fast, but fast enough to be ahead of my age-group challengers. I was, as usual, being overtaken, but not by my age group, and this was a great motivation. I pushed my legs as hard as I could muster, and the downpour seemed to distract me from the pain. I loved the last 100 metres of the run leg, giving it my all as I powered up the blue carpet with the spectators shouting my name.

On finishing the race, and without even stopping to pick up my finishing medal, I went into the first aid tent and asked for help cleaning up my injuries.

The mixture of adrenaline and endorphins clearly had an amazing effect on me: even though the gouges on my knee and elbow were deep and looked nasty, I could still feel no pain. (I knew it was going to be very sore later, though.) I asked the paramedics to be as brutal as they needed to be to get out all the gravel while I couldn't feel it.

It had been such an eventful race, and one that I will never forget. Such trials sum up the challenges experienced by a triathlete – from the calming experience of swimming alongside the jellyfish to finding the inner strength that enabled me to carry on despite facing serious physical challenges.

The fall was a shock, but it helped me learn a useful lesson about getting up and getting on with it, and to know that in a race and in the heat of competition, an injury doesn't hurt like it would in normal life.

When I collected my race results, I found that I had surpassed myself. For the first time, I was top of my age group. I had smashed the swim, knocking more than a minute off my personal best; my bike was fast; and even with the numb foot and injuries, I had managed to post my second fastest 5-kilometre run, with a time of 26 minutes, 5 seconds.

I went home battered and bandaged, yet very happy. My triathlon adventure was presenting me with so many unexpected challenges – and I was overcoming them.

CHAPTER 17

SWIMMING LIKE A SHARK

'I was ready to race. What I wasn't ready for were the sharp elbows.'

'It's all right for you, you come from a swimming background!'

I often get that comment from my fellow triathletes as we shiver nervously, standing next to each other and wrapped in matching neoprene, looking out over the water before a race, and it always makes me laugh.

It sounds like I have competed in the Olympic Games and won a ton of medals. The truth is far from that: I gave up swimming competitively when I was 15, and never won a medal for my county, let alone my country.

They are right in another sense, though: swimming seems to be a part of my DNA. Family legend has it that I could swim before I could walk.

I was born in Victoria Barracks in the heart of Hong Kong in the middle of Typhoon Shirley. My father was an Irish Guards officer serving in the British Army as aide-de-camp to the Commander British Forces. I spent my first couple of years living in a flat at the top of Garden Mansions, a 20-storey high-rise in Repulse Bay. In those days, 20 stories was quite tall, though it would be dwarfed in the Hong Kong of the 21st century with its tightly packed skyscrapers.

One of my first memories involves a love of water. I was sitting in the bath while there was an almighty storm going on outside and typhoon-strength winds. I remember being quite unconcerned, mesmerised by the bathwater swilling from side to side as the building swayed in the winds. Scary as it sounds, high-rise buildings are designed to move and sway; otherwise, they would collapse under the pressure.

Later, we moved to a house, an army quarter on the tip of Stanley Peninsula with stunning views over the vast expanse of the South China Sea. It was an amazing place to grow up and we would find and catch poisonous snakes in the garden. We also adopted our first pet, a tiny little fluffy mongrel called Mali, who was found sitting under my father's desk in Army HQ and refused to leave.

Because we lived in such a hot humid climate, my parents would take me swimming as often as possible, either in a pool or, if we were especially lucky, out on the sea on the General's junk. A junk is a wooden sailing boat with fully battened sails – the same design as the sailing ships first used by the Chinese for trading in the second century.

I was so tiny I would be harnessed into my cot at the front of the boat, the wind blowing in my short blonde hair as we headed out over the bright blue waters to catch the cooler breeze.

It was on these journeys that I made my first forays into the water. Mum and Dad would put a pair of bright orange armbands on me, and then throw me high into the air from the boat, into the water below. I would land with a huge splash, laughing with the excitement. They say their friends were horrified at the sight of it, but I really loved it, and wanted to be thrown in over and over again.

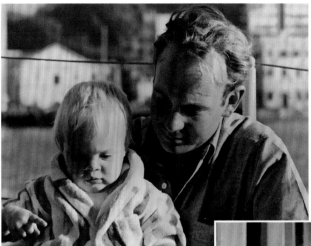

◀ Wrapped up warm after a swim with my Dad in Hong Kong, where he was serving as an Irish Guards Officer in the British Army.

▼ Full 1980s fashion, aged 15, around the time I sadly gave up competitive swimming because I thought it made me look too muscly.

▼ On one of the rare occasions I wore armbands, about to launch myself into a pool. You can clearly see the joy on my face and how much I loved it.

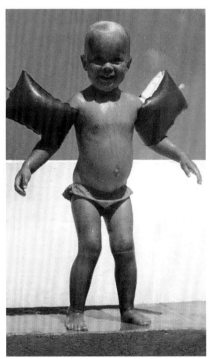

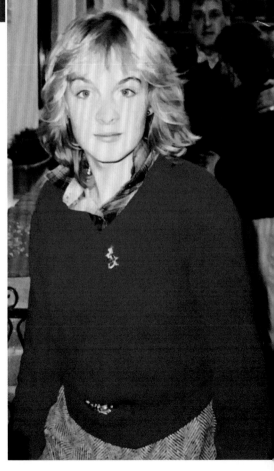

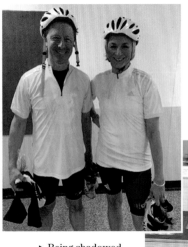

◄ I love this picture and it makes me laugh, as neither Charlie nor I had worn Lycra or cycling shoes before, and as you can see we were both utterly clueless. This was taken just before my life-changing race at the Manchester Velodrome in December 2012.

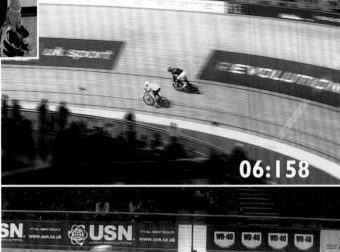

▶ Being shadowed by Olympic gold medallist Ed Clancy, as I raced around the Manchester Velodrome for the *BBC Breakfast* Christmas Challenge.

▶ A life-changing 23 seconds – the moment I crossed the finish line at the *BBC Breakfast* Christmas Challenge. Thankfully since then I have improved my cycling style.

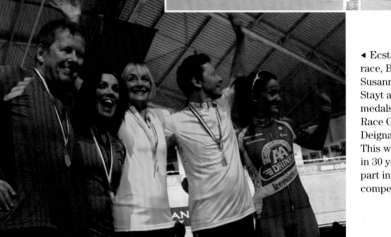

◄ Ecstatic after the race, Bill Turnbull, Susanna Reid, Charlie Stayt and I are given our medals by World Road Race Champion Lizzie Deignan, née Armitstead. This was the first time in 30 years I had taken part in any form of competitive sport.

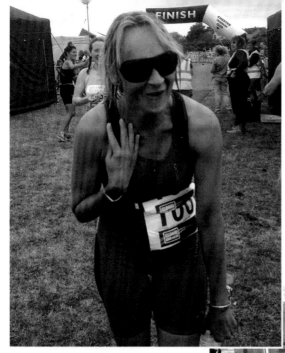

◄ Smiling but in pain with an agonising stitch after finishing my first ever triathlon, with the Deva Divas in my home city, Chester, in July 2013.

► The best of both worlds. Interviewing top triathlete Jonathan Brownlee, Olympic silver medalist at the World Championships in Rotterdam, with Paul Redgrove on cameras.

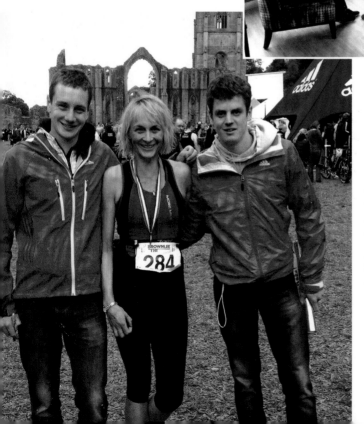

◄ With two of my triathlon heroes, Olympic gold and silver medallists Alistair and Jonathan Brownlee. This photograph was taken after I finished the Brownlee Tri at Fountains Abbey in Yorkshire, in September 2013.

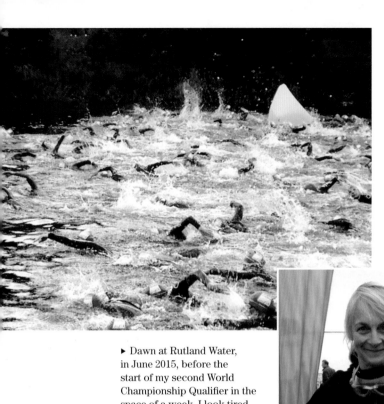

◄ I'm the one in the red swimming cap! The intimidating washing machine of swimmers at the start of my first World Championship Qualifier, the Deva Triathlon in Chester, in 2015.

▶ Dawn at Rutland Water, in June 2015, before the start of my second World Championship Qualifier in the space of a week. I look tired but determined to try again

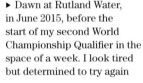

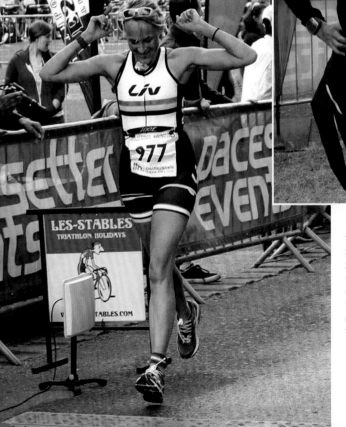

◄ I didn't know it then, but this was the moment I qualified for the World Championships, embarrassingly wearing two triathlon suits as I had failed to pack a sports bra!

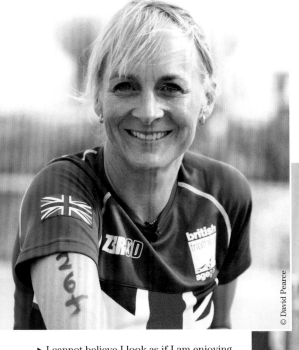

◄ The realisation of what seemed to be an impossible dream… I was about to represent Great Britain in my age-group in the triathlon World Championships in Chicago in 2015.

© David Pearce

▶ I cannot believe I look as if I am enjoying myself in this photo, because at the time I felt like I was running through sand without an ounce of energy!

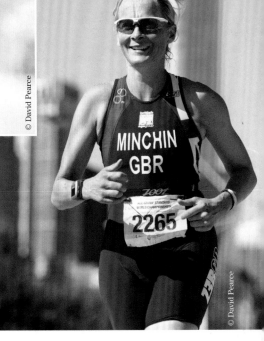

© David Pearce

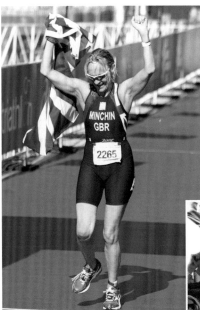

◄ The finishing line. I had tripped over the flag in my hand only seconds before this photo was taken but just managed to hold myself together.

▶ One of my proudest moments, taking part in the Parade of Nations at sunset by Buckingham Fountain, Chicago, with dozens of other GB age-groupers.

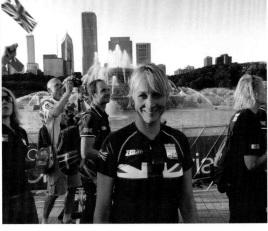

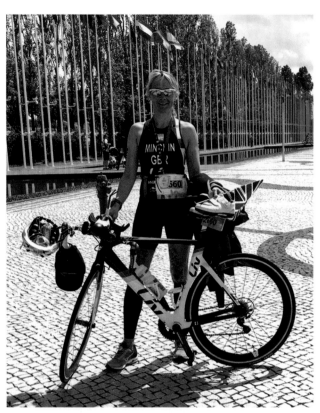

◄ Four years since my first triathlon, at the European Championships in Lisbon in June 2016, and I finally look like I know what I am doing. You can see the medical tape on my injured knee.

▼ This girl can, and these girls can. The joy, excitement and anticipation in this picture before the swim at the Liverpool Tri is palpable.

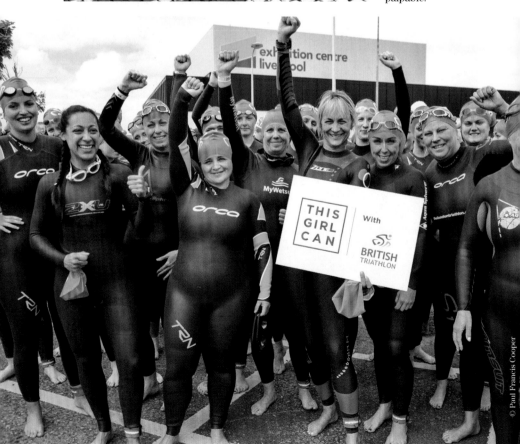

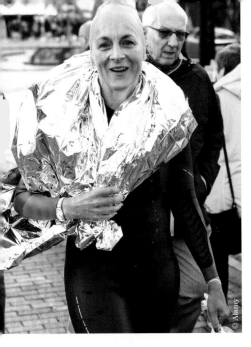

◄ Over the years I have competed in dozens of different races. This was after swimming a mile in Salford Quays, just outside the *BBC Breakfast* studios.

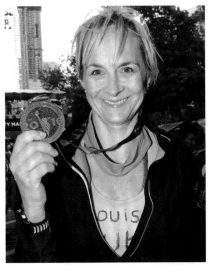

▲ Holding my medal proudly at the end of the hardest run ever, the New York City Marathon in November 2016. Two minutes later I was overcome with emotion and burst into inconsolable tears.

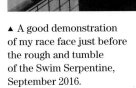

▲ A good demonstration of my race face just before the rough and tumble of the Swim Serpentine, September 2016.

► I love relays, and this was one of my favourites, the mixed-relay at Cholmomdeley Castle in Cheshire in 2017.

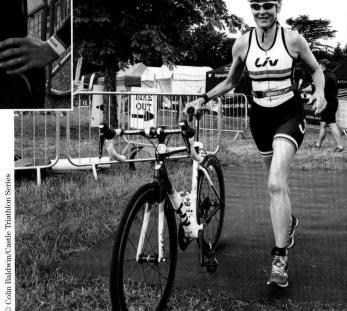

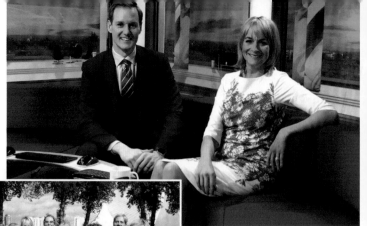

► Where I spend early mornings, at work with my co-host Dan Walker, on the famous *BBC Breakfast* red sofa.

◄ Surrounded by the awesome athletes from the GB age-group team in Rotterdam, September 2017.

▼ Looking nervous just before the World Championships in Rotterdam, surrounded by gear and going through last minute checks. I have raced dozens of times but as you can see I still get nervous.

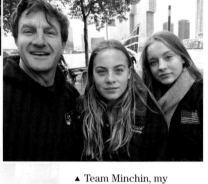

▲ Team Minchin, my wonderful and dedicated supporters: David, Scarlett and Mia, at the World Championships in Rotterdam, September 2017.

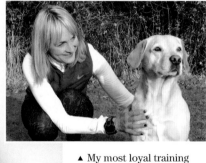

▲ My most loyal training partner, Waffle, who has never once let me down.

Aged just two, I ditched the armbands. Apparently, right from the start I swam without fear and with a total affinity for the water: eyes wide open, kicking ferociously, and every now and then surfacing for a breath. I would spend hours in the water, and I remember being furious every time I had to get out. Being totally immersed or floating peacefully on the surface seemed to be the most natural place to me – much easier than trying to toddle about on hot, humid land.

I continued to love swimming when we moved back to the UK. Even though the pools in Bracknell Leisure Centre were very different from the South China Sea, I would swim as often as my mother would take me. She hated every minute of it, but she knew I loved it, so she dragged herself into the hot, steamy atmosphere, and dutifully tried to help my brother swim in the children's pool while my sister, Nikki, and I were off in the deep pool, racing up and down – and, to the horror of the lifeguards, seeing how long we could hold our breath underwater at the bottom.

Mum's dedication was rewarded every summer with peace and quiet. My grandparents had retired to live in Javea near Alicante in Spain, where they had a house up on the hills with a tiny oval swimming pool. Every summer, we spent two glorious weeks staying with them, and Mum could sit by the pool covered in baby lotion to improve her tan, and only vaguely watching because she knew we were safe swimming. We spent every waking hour splashing about and playing endless games in the water. By the end of the fortnight, our hair had turned bright green with the chlorine. The only time we would dry off was at siesta time, when my grandparents would drag us out and make us have a couple of quiet hours lying down. I think it was to give themselves a break!

One of the things I most looked forward to on those holidays was our forays to the beach. My grandmother made us sandwiches out of soft white bread, which would gradually be soaked in the juice of the ripe tomatoes packed inside them, and we then headed down to the coast. I always raced my cousins to the beach, determined to be the first to dive straight into the warm water. Being in the sea was exhilarating: you could go from floating in flat calm one moment to being rocked the next by enormous sets of waves that caught you, dragged you under and tumbled you about like a wet towel in a washing machine. In the blind panic of being crushed by gallons of water, I wouldn't know which way was up, but would always eventually pop to the surface, gasping for air and laughing hysterically at the terror of it.

I remember one day happily swimming with my sister, Nikki, far out of our depth and seeing the terrifying sight of a huge set of waves marching towards us. They were much bigger than I had ever seen before, and I knew that we would be in serious trouble if they broke over us. It was too late for us to reach the safety of the beach, so I shouted: 'It will be OK, follow me!' to Nikki, and we swam straight out to sea towards them. From our vantage point, we looked back to see my parents aghast on the beach as the waves crashed, searching anxiously in the surf for us while we floated harmlessly over the top of the waves on gentle unbroken water.

I learned to swim without any formal lessons, and picked up most of my technique from watching my dad, who was a wonderfully fast and graceful swimmer. I remember an idyllic summer when he spent hours on the edge of the pool, patiently teaching me how to dive in. I started sitting with my bottom on the poolside, arms aloft, hands together and toppling myself in. I eventually graduated to standing and diving in. Dozens of painful bellyflops later, I could pull off quite a convincing racing start.

My memory of my first real swimming race is still very clear. When I think about it, my heart beats faster.

I was in primary school in Wokingham, Berkshire, and the pool was minuscule, maybe only 10 metres long. I was racing against a girl who was two years above me and about a foot taller than me. Because she was so tall, all she had to do to beat me was make sure she did a good dive, then add just a couple of strokes and she would virtually touch the other end.

As I lined up at the pool's edge, I thought that the odds were stacked against me and I didn't have the slightest chance. But as the whistle blew, I sprang into life, did a racing dive, and swam like mad. To my shock, and to the astonishment of most people watching, who had assumed she would win because she was so tall, I beat her by about a metre and went home proudly holding the school swimming cup.

After that, the trips to the swimming pool in Bracknell took on a more serious tone. Mum signed me up for a swimming club, and I joined in endless drills up and down the lanes with dozens of other young swimmers. I could just about keep up with them, but having never had a lesson in my life, my technique was seriously lacking and my first swimming gala was a disaster.

When we arrived, the air in the pool was hot, and the atmosphere close and overpowering. The noise from the loud-speakers and the parents cheering was deafening. I had never raced before, so I didn't even know how to dive off one of the blocks. I watched the other more experienced children, and tried to copy them.

I had been entered for a breaststroke race. That was my least favourite stroke, so I wasn't feeling very confident, but I raced well in the first couple of heats and made it through to the finals. We waited for what seemed to be hours for the deciding race. Excitingly for me, that was way past my bedtime. All being well, and if I could hold my pace, I might be in with the chance of a medal.

I swam as hard as I possibly could, giving every single ounce of energy – and touched the side in third place! The family were leaping about in excitement and I was thrilled. My first medal! How exciting.

My joy was to be short-lived, though. I could see two of the officials pointing at me and having an intense discussion, which filled me with dread. What had I done wrong? They came over to me and broke the bad news: 'You have been disqualified.'

Disqualified? For what? Had I cheated? They explained to me that I had used an illegal kick. The breaststroke rules say that your legs should move simultaneously, each a mirror image of the other. I was swimming lopsided. I was devastated because I had no idea I had been doing it. Without ever having had a lesson, I had been swimming slightly wrong. I went home wet, tired and dispirited.

By the time I went to secondary school, I had learned how to kick properly. In the summer terms, I trained at every opportunity I could. I spent endless happy hours in the pool pacing up and down, perfecting my technique.

Very soon, I started representing the school. I raced alongside a friend, who was also an excellent swimmer. We won every race we entered. The only ones we didn't win were the relays, when we needed other people in the team. It was a golden time and I loved everything about it – the training, the racing and, of course, the winning.

Then, at about the age of 15, I decided I had had enough.

Like so many teenage girls, I had become increasingly self-conscious and uncomfortable about how I looked. Instead of celebrating my powerful, muscly shoulders, as I do now, I had begun to think they made me look unfeminine. So, very suddenly, I stopped swimming altogether. I stopped entering races and I stopped the training.

I look back now and think what a terrible shame that was. I had loved swimming so much, and it was such an important and fun part of my life, especially in the difficult period of trying to navigate my way into adulthood and through a whole series of important exams. Curiously, though, I didn't miss it at all at the time.

Stopping so suddenly, and right at the top of my game, had a couple of curious effects on me.

Firstly, I had become so accustomed to never being beaten in a swimming race that the thought of losing filled me with dread. I still loved swimming and on holiday would spend hours in the sea or in the pool, but if anyone suggested a race, even for fun, I would refuse. It didn't matter who was asking, I just couldn't countenance the thought of being beaten by anyone, so I always made up some ridiculous excuse not to take part. If ever I was forced to take part, I tried to look like I didn't care, but inside my heart was beating as fast as it had before a school race, and I swam as if my life depended on it.

The second consequence of giving up so early is with me even now. Wherever I am swimming, whether in a pool or in open water, I can't help myself: if I see someone come up alongside to overtake me, I put in a burst of speed. That has resulted in lots of hilariously competitive incidents, mostly involving men. I imagine they are thinking, 'Look at her, she thinks she is swimming fast, I can definitely overtake her'.

To my immense and childish satisfaction, most of them can't – unless I am trying to stick to a particularly slow set of lengths, which Claire, my coach, has planned for me. Even then, I can't stop myself from racing. As soon as I catch sight of someone swimming well beside me, my swimming accelerator ignites. I kick as hard as I can, at maximum speed, and even if I am broken at the end of the length I always breathe quietly and pretend it has been no effort at all!

The most embarrassing time I succumbed to the racing bug was in open water in Manley Mere in Cheshire. In the summer I often go to train there. I was about 600 metres round the 750-metre course when I could see on my left an incredibly fast swimmer moving alongside to overtake me. Obviously I wasn't having that, so I dug in, put my head down and, as fast as I could, raced for the beach.

I think we just about arrived there together. I was seriously out of breath but trying not to show it, when I realised, to my horror, that I had been racing against my swimming coach, Chris Malpass. Chris competed for Team GB as a junior, has held numerous British Masters records, and is regularly ranked in the Top 10 in the world in Masters swimming. The bottom line is, he is a top-level swimmer, and I had basically challenged him to a race.

What did I think I was doing? He just laughed and said, 'I should have guessed that was you!' Then he delighted in telling me that he was just finishing his seventh time round the lake. I had been on my first, so my fresh set of arms was the only reason I had been able to keep up!

My stupidly competitive approach to swimming does sometimes work to my advantage, however. In the summer of 2016, the organisers behind the London Marathon held a swimming festival in Hyde Park, which had been the venue for the open-water swimming at the 2012 Olympics. It was a mass participation event and thousands of swimmers descended to swim a mile in the Serpentine. For logistical reasons, I could only swim in the final wave. Competitors had to get around the course in a particularly tight finish time, so the lake was full of very fast and mostly male swimmers.

Normally, in a triathlon, I swim in a women's-only wave. They can be quite feisty, with arms and legs everywhere, but no one is bashing you on purpose. Besides, I like to give people the benefit of the doubt, and assume that they can't see where I am anyway.

Not so in my race in the Serpentine!

After a couple of minutes of warm-up, I could see that people were taking it very seriously. Having done so many races before, I wasn't intimidated. I was ready to race. What I wasn't ready for were the sharp elbows.

From the off, it was like being tumbled in those waves in Spain all over again. There were people swimming over me, grabbing at my legs, hanging on to my feet, scrabbling at my goggles, pulling me under. I was floundering, gasping for breath, and praying that after a few minutes it would stop. It didn't and I was still being bashed about after 500 metres, when I reached the turnaround point towards Hyde Park Corner. I just couldn't believe it, and thought, *This is absurd. I don't want to race like this. I am just going to stop.* That lasted a couple of seconds before my swimming racing demon piped up. *No, you are not going to stop. You are just going to get on with it and swim faster.*

It was like I had switched on a turbocharger. I swam like a shark down the long stretch of water by the side of the lido, didn't slow down when I turned around the last buoys and sprinted towards the large floating jetty to reach my hand up and touch the finish line. I was closely followed by another woman, wearing a matching yellow hat, which meant she was in the same wave as me. She made me laugh when she said with a huge smile, 'Ha, we really chicked them, didn't we?'

It was the first time anyone had ever said that to me, but I knew exactly what she meant as I watched a stream of men wearing yellow hats get out of the water long after us. I checked my results and was delighted to see that the added pressure, and my racing demon, had knocked a whole minute off my 1-mile personal best. I had finished the race in 25 minutes, 49 seconds, coming fifth in the 40+ age group.

Not bad for an afternoon swim in the park.

CHAPTER 18

LET THE WORLD CHAMPIONSHIPS BEGIN

'We had been competing against each other, but now we were racing together and there was an infectious sense of camaraderie.'

Finally, in September 2015, the moment for which I had been training arrived. We touched down in Chicago, the Windy City, ahead of the World Triathlon Championships.

I was so excited. After 18 months of relentless training and racing, while juggling the logistics of home life and getting up at an unearthly hour to present *BBC Breakfast*, I had made it. I was in Chicago, along with 450 other age-groupers from the Great Britain team, ready to race against athletes from all over the world.

David, Mia and Scarlett, my most loyal supporters for all this time, were determined not to miss out. They had flown out to be there with me, and were joined by my dad, Patrick, and my younger brother, Mark.

We were staying in the main hotel for the Great Britain team, the iconic Renaissance Blackstone. I was delighted to find that staying there too was my fellow Chester Tri Club triathlete Sharon Plested. She had been with me all the way along my triathlon qualification journey, and I always loved racing with her. She was in the age group above me and faster than I was, and she had been a constant source of advice, help and reassurance.

The hotel was situated right in the heart of Chicago on South Michigan Avenue, which turned out to be in a fantastic location right next to the course. It offered stunning views of the bright blue waters of Lake Michigan, as well as the bike route for the triathlon and the running course.

Right from the start, it was wonderful to be part of the team.

Everyone was proudly wearing the GB kit and there was constant chatter in the lifts and the lobby – about what was happening outside, as well as snippets of race news and information.

One of the highlights for me was taking part in the opening ceremony beside Lake Michigan. I have always loved watching the Parade of Nations in the Opening Ceremony of the Olympic Games and I couldn't believe that now I was taking part in something very similar.

The event was bathed in a warm orange evening sunshine, and as dozens of national flags fluttered I felt incredibly proud and privileged. Great Britain, along with the US, had by far the biggest number of competing triathletes, and we all spent a wonderful hour or so laughing and waving as we paraded around the Buckingham Fountain while supporters cheered from the grandstands.

BBC Breakfast had sent a camera crew to Chicago consisting of our Planning Editor, Lisa Kelly, and cameraman Brijesh Patel to film my triathlon experience. Before we flew to America, Lisa had been in touch with the other nine or so women competing for Great Britain in my age group, and had arranged for six of us to meet up on Olive Park Beach, to have a chat and then swim together.

All of my fellow competitors were just as excited as I was to be there, and it was inspiring to stand beside them, on the hot white sand, dressed in our matching GB tri suits. In the months running up to the World Championships, we had been competing against each other, but now we were racing together and there was an infectious sense of camaraderie.

The feeling was echoed in the whole city, which seemed to have been invaded by triathletes. Everywhere you walked you would be overtaken by gaggles of athletes dressed in their home strips from all over the world – Mexico, Spain, France, Germany, and so on. You couldn't move for triathletes: they were jogging along the pavements, running by the lakeside or out on their sleek racing bikes trying out the route. It was like being part of a gigantic triathlon festival. Except, of course, that this was a festival where everyone was shunning alcohol and instead opting for energy drinks and gels.

There was so much to watch and look forward to in the run-up to my race, including the Men's and Women's World Championships and the Paratriathlon World Championships. The elite course was different to ours: both the bike and the run route consisted of several loops up and down Lake Shore Drive and Columbus Drive, parallel to Lake Michigan.

From a spectator point of view, it was intoxicating. If you stood on the pavement, you could get a close-up of the elite athletes hustling their way through the race. I watched in awe as Non Stanford and Vicky Holland worked together to push hard on the cycle route, and came second and third behind the incredible American triathlete Gwen Jorgensen. The race was especially exciting because their places on the podium meant that they secured their Olympic qualifications.

Watching these elite triathletes inspired me and gave me even more of a sense of occasion. I was going to be racing on parts of the same course as them. And with a bit of luck, I would run down the same blue carpet to the finish.

CHAPTER 19

A DREAM FULFILLED?

'Each group of supporters was like a tiny island of hope in a sea of hot tarmac.'

The most important day of my triathlon career started very early with an alarming jolt. At 2 a.m., screeching alarms simultaneously blasted from David's and my own mobile phones.

I scrabbled about for my mobile, trying not to wake up Mia and Scarlett, who were sleeping soundly on the other side of the room. Squinting in the darkness at the ungodly hour, I read an alarming message: Imminent Threat Alert. The message had been sent by the National Weather Service to warn us that there was a dangerous storm on the way, one that was a potential threat to life, and we were to take cover!

Stumbling over to the window to check the streets below, I looked towards Lake Michigan and could see the huge trees bent over, battered by the wind and driving rain. I hoped that 'taking cover' meant staying in our hotel bedroom, shuddering at the thought that I was supposed to be racing on those rain-soaked streets in only a matter of hours.

At the time, I had no idea how the text got through to us. Later, I discovered it was a Wireless Emergency Alert, an efficient system of mass notification used to warn the public about danger. Only the President, state and public health officials, the National Weather Service and the National Center for Missing and Exploited Children can send these short emergency messages, which go to all mobile devices in a specific geographic area. There is no need to subscribe to the messages; they override the network. So if you are in the vicinity in danger and your phone is on, you will get the alert. It is so loud – and unlike any other sound on a mobile – that there is no way to miss it.

The message had been sent to hundreds of thousands of people in the area, so I was by no means the only triathlete whose sleep had been disturbed.

Such was the alarming shock of the message, there was no way I could go back to sleep. My restless brain started playing tricks on me. I began to have serious misgivings about the day's race. *What am I doing? Why am I taking part in a serious race with world champions? How will I overcome my nerves and even start it, let alone finish? What if the swim is really tough and I panic like I did in my first triathlon? What if my bike gets a puncture? What if I fall off my bike and hurt myself? What if I just can't run?* Endless doomsday scenarios played in a loop in my head.

If that wasn't bad enough, another thought also plagued me. We had filmed a preview of the race when we arrived in Chicago, and this had been shown on *BBC Breakfast* that morning – which meant that millions of loyal viewers now knew exactly what I was trying to do. *What if I fail? Will I fail them too? How will I be able to go back to the famous red* Breakfast *sofa, head held high, if I don't even finish?*

To try to distract myself, I started reading the dozens of tweets of encouragement from family, friends and *Breakfast* viewers who had been messaging me overnight, offering me support in my mad endeavour. 'Go Louise.' 'You are brilliant.' 'What an inspiration.' 'You can do this.' I had been inundated with goodwill messages, and after reading them, I finally calmed down and devised a simple race plan.

First, I gave myself a few reminders. I had spent more than a year trying incredibly hard, dedicating hours to training and racing, making incremental and painful steps – and all the hard work, dedication and determination had paid off. I had done it, I had made it, I was in the Great Britain triathlon team, I was at the World Championships. That had been the goal when I sat down with my coach, Claire, about a year ago. Here I was, in Chicago, with my kit saying Minchin GBR: I was a bona fide member of the team. I came to the conclusion that all the pressure was off. There was no need to race for a particular time. I didn't need to beat anyone; I didn't even need to get a personal best. All I had to do was enjoy the experience, do my best on the day, and get across the finish line safely. It was a huge relief to realise that the time didn't matter, just that I finished what I had set out to do.

With my new 'race safely' plan in my head, I finally fell asleep for a couple of hours before my alarm went off. The ferocious storm had passed through and Chicago looked clean, new and washed by the rain.

As ever on competition day, and even at that early hour, there were butterflies in my stomach. I had laid out everything I would need for the race the night before, and now went through my scribbled checklist. Carefully I packed into my backpack my cycle shoes, trainers, talcum powder to sprinkle in my shoes (making them easier to put on in a rush), energy gels and tablets, sunglasses and water.

Thankfully, all of us triathletes who were staying in the hotel had been allowed to keep our bikes in our bedrooms. I gave it a quick once-over, checked the tyre pressures and wheeled it down the corridor. Dozens of fellow triathletes were on their way, clogging up the lifts, and I had to lift my bike upright on its back wheel, squeezing it into the lift vertically.

Outside, the temperature had dropped considerably. I was shivering as I cycled towards transition, only a short distance from the hotel, crossing the wide bridge over the railway tracks and towards Lake Michigan.

When I arrived, I saw where we were going to rack our bikes – and my heart sank. I had assumed that our transition would match the transitions for the elite athletes competing on the world stage: a pristine blue carpet, shiny metal bike racks neatly lined up in uniform rows, and large, clear numbers marking each competitor's position. The reality couldn't have been more different, or more disappointing. Transition was a muddy, scrubby piece of land, on a slight hill, with patches of sand where the grass had been worn away. Not what I had imagined for the World Triathlon Championships.

Snazzy bikes, more than I had ever seen, were all jammed together there in one place. Pinarellos, Giants, Specialized, Cannondales and Cervélos, with carbon frames, disc wheels, racing tyres and aerobars, all thoughtfully designed to make their riders as fast as possible.

Security was tight – partly, I imagine, because of the price of the bikes. When I reached the front of the queue the guard inspected my kitbag, as well as the back of my calf, looking for the F45 scrawled there in indelible ink by officials when I had registered the day before. This meant I was in the Female 45–50 category.

I was let through, and it took me a couple of minutes to work out where my bike was going to be racked. Luckily my rack was the furthest to the left – a relief, since this would at least make it easy to find when I was running back into transition in my wetsuit after the swim.

Lisa and Brij were already buzzing about transition, busy filming in their hi-vis jackets. As I organised myself, I tried not to get distracted by the camera rolling. I hooked my bike's saddle on to the metal bar on top of my number, 2225. This was a bit tricky because the bikes were closely packed together with only about a 30cm gap between each one. The tight squeeze meant I had to be very precise about how I laid out my cycle shoes and running shoes in the small space under my bike. I made sure my helmet was balanced carefully on my tri bars with the straps open and undone, so there was no way I would get distracted and touch my bike before I put my helmet on. Hopefully this would rule out the possibility of a disqualification.

As I had learned, I Sellotaped a spare contact lens to my bike frame, just in case one fell out in the swim, and three of my favourite energy jelly sweets to the bar.

Next, I juggled two bottles of water in my hands. Thinking I was cold, foolishly imagining that it would be a similar temperature at 1 p.m. when I raced, and arguing that I had never yet finished a 750-millilitre bottle on the 40-kilometre bike leg, I decided that I didn't need the extra weight of carrying two full bottles. A poor decision, but I had no idea. I put just one bottle in the cage on the bike frame, and left a tiny screw-top water bottle next to my shoes, just in case.

Checking that my transition area looked the same as everyone else's, I felt calm and well prepared, then headed back out to while away the time before the start. I took one last look at my bike, trying to memorise where it was – far left, middle of the rack – when I saw my fellow Chester Tri Club member Sharon Plested walking towards me with her bike. We had raced together so many times during qualifying year, and she had always been a great support. Routinely passing me on the run leg, she was always ready to shout encouragement like: 'Come on, Minchin, you can do this!'

On World Championship Race day, though, she was overcome by the occasion, tearful and ashen with fear. I hugged her and promised that it would all be OK.

The waiting before the start on race-day is always the worst bit for me. My tummy rumbles, my nerves jangle, I can't think straight, I can't remember where anything is, I imagine that I have forgotten something crucial and, most irritatingly of all, I am unable to hold any sort of conversation. David, Mia and Scarlett are always brilliant at dealing with it, and take absolutely no nonsense. When I start saying things like *I don't want to get into the water, I am never going to finish, what am I doing, and why I am here anyway?*, they tell me to be quiet, stop being so silly and just get on with it.

On that day, to make things worse, the 45–50 age group was one of the last waves of the day to start. As I paced up and down the shoreline in my wetsuit, watching wave after wave of different age groups jump off the pontoon to start their 1,500-metre swim, the aquamarine waters of Lake Michigan were becoming increasingly choppy. We were meant to set off at 12.40 p.m., but the athletes due to start before us were being delayed, and the start times were starting to slip.

I wasn't worried about the swell. Swimming was my strongest discipline, and having had lots of practice in open water and the waves off the North Cornish coast I believed that the worsening conditions would be an advantage. The bigger the waves, the better. What's more, lots of my fellow athletes would be put off, giving me the chance to make a fast start and get ahead of them on the bike.

Then, unbelievably, just as we were about to go into the pre-race holding pen and with only minutes before the whistle, officials announced that the pontoon had come off its moorings. It was too dangerous to start from there and so, for safety reasons, they were going to change the course! Instead of a distance of 1,500 metres, it would be only 750 metres. I was hugely disappointed. Any advantage I might have had was immediately halved. I didn't let this worry me, though: less time in the water meant less time for things to go wrong, which played into my safe race plan.

To have any chance of getting a good swim under my belt, I knew I had to be brave, take my heart in my hands and start as close to the front as I could. I made my way purposefully right to the front of the 70 or so women in my race. If all went well, and I got a good start, I wouldn't get stuck in the now familiar but still daunting washing-machine of triathletes kicking, splashing and thrashing their way through the lake.

I waved one last goodbye to my family, took a breath and was third to jump straight into the deep water. The sharp cold took my breath away, but I swam away from the shore to the left-hand side to give myself some extra space, away from all the elbows. My teammate Morag McDowall was close behind me into the water, and we now chatted nervously about strategy while we watched everyone else leaping in. She was so encouraging, but I knew that she was nervous about the swim, so I told her to get right behind me and see if she could take advantage of the draft I would make through the water.

The course was now effectively a straight line horizontally along the harbour wall, which should have been easy to navigate. The size of the waves, which seemed much bigger now we were all bobbing about in them, meant that I couldn't see the huge yellow buoys marking the right-hand turn to the exit. Far in the distance I spotted a white building, which I now know was the Shedd Aquarium, so I decided to head towards it, assuming that eventually I would find the way out and back to transition.

I tried to calm my racing heart during the wait for the countdown. Suddenly the klaxon blared and we were off. The race had begun. No time to think any more, this was it: I had to swim as fast and as straight as possible. There was a bit of bashing from some of the other swimmers as we tried to make space, but after the first 100 metres I was exactly where I wanted to be: near the front.

Settling into a fast and smooth front crawl, I tried to calm my breathing, and looked up every couple of strokes to check I was going in the right direction. It was still difficult to see where we were heading, and I thought the easiest thing to do was to keep close to the sea wall. If I did that, and kept up the pace, I would eventually get there. It was then that I started to hear cheering. When I looked up on my next stroke I caught a glimpse of my family. There they were: David, Mia, Scarlett, Dad and Mark, walking beside me like angels, cheering me on. I gave them such a broad smile I swallowed a mouthful of water.

The course had been halved, but it still felt tough. I struggled through the waves and weeds, trying my best to catch sight of the finish. My goggles steamed up, making it even more difficult to see the end, but I caught a glimpse of a few swimmers ahead and was reassured that at least a couple of others were swimming in the same direction. The visibility was so bad that I almost bumped into two enormous buoys marking the exit, but I did a sharp right on to the blue-carpeted ramp, and was hauled out by the safe hands of an official up on to my feet.

'Great swim,' shouted my brother, Mark, who had been watching and waiting for me, and his presence was a massive boost to my confidence. I gave him a cheery wave and a smile as I tore off my goggles and swimming hat and started out on the 500-metre run towards my bike. On the way I passed Maria Powell, the best British swimmer in our age group. She had exited the water ahead of me, but she was injured and was walking along the route. I arrived into transition and quickly found my bike, excited to see that most of my age group's bicycles were still racked and waiting for their riders. I wasn't alone, though. Fellow GB triathlete Anita Howe had caught up with me, and her bike was right next to mine, but we were both breathing too hard to talk, and concentrating on the race.

I had practised a fast transition from swim to cycle, and now went into automatic pilot, dragging off my wetsuit, stepping on it to get my feet out, throwing it in a heap under the bike, fastening my shoes, clipping on my helmet, swallowing an energy gel, then finally wheeling my bike, hand on the seat, as speedily as possible to the mount line.

The cycle route was a 40-kilometre double loop. First, it headed north up the wide expanse of South Columbus Drive towards Trump Tower and the Chicago Loop. Next it led down a steep incline underground on to Lower Wacker Drive, an impressive but labyrinthine triple-decker expressway that you may remember seeing in *The Blues Brothers*; the fabulously over-the-top police car chase was filmed there. It then headed back south again on Columbus Drive, descending on to the McCormick Place Busway, crossing over the railway tracks a couple of times, round a sharp turn and all the way back. All the roads were closed to traffic and it was a fast but very technical course, with lots of tricky bends and dead turns.

I was so excited to be out on my bike, and felt great whizzing along in the glorious sunshine. The first circuit was fantastic: I was making great progress and gave Lisa and Brij, who were filming, an exuberant wave as I sped past them. The other teammates in my age group soon caught me up, though. The first to overtake me was dynamo Mo, about three kilometres from the start, and then, in quick succession, Mel Clarke, Maria Powell, Ceri Cook and Lisa Williams.

I was fine with that. Just being out on the course with them was great fun. My aim had been to have a safe and successful race. But just before I started the second lap, things started to go wrong. It was now extremely hot, the sun was beginning to burn, and I had run out of water, finishing the whole bottle only halfway through the ride. I was already very thirsty, and there were another 20 kilometres still left to go. Very soon my mind started playing tricks. As I rode into the darkness of the subterranean Wacker Drive, it felt like the heat was pressing down on me and the walls were closing in. To add to the growing sense of claustrophobia, there were no other cyclists in sight – for 10 long, panicky minutes. I started to think that I had completely messed up, wasn't even on the course any more, and would never find the way out.

I stuck with it, though, and my fright made me speed up. Eventually I caught up with another cyclist. It was a relief to have another rider in sight, although they soon pulled away as we went up the steep ramp back into the baking Chicago sunshine. The lack of water was now also sapping my energy and slowing me down. I tried an energy jelly sweet to boost my strength, but my mouth was so dry I couldn't face eating more than one.

My brother Mark had done a brilliant recce of the course and had managed to scope out about six different vantage points to cheer me on. I was incredibly relieved to hear him and Mia shouting my name as I cycled back on the busway. On my return, they were there again, to shout encouragement, leaning over the bridge, waving madly and cheering me on.

My raging thirst was all I could think about. When I remembered I had left that small screw-top bottle of water in transition, I fixated on it. Make my way back to transition without collapsing, and I could down it in one. No longer so dehydrated, I could then try to get my race back into some semblance of order.

As I negotiated the last dead turn and cycled towards the dismount line, David was waiting for me behind the safety barriers. 'Slow down!' he shouted. I could see why he was concerned. A Mexican athlete, who must have been in my age group, was gingerly picking herself up from the floor after coming in too fast and falling off her bike. Ouch.

Safety was not my priority, though. I was desperate for a drink.

This time, my transition preparation paid off. Exactly as I had been taught to, I had run from the entrance to the exit several times before leaving for the start of the race, so I now easily found my wetsuit and running shoes. I assumed my thirst problem would be over in a second. I quickly racked my bike and made a grab for my tiny bottle of water. As I unscrewed the lid, I was shaking with adrenaline and exertion. My hands were trembling so badly that I dropped the bottle and could only watch, helpless, as every single drop of water spilled on to the grass and sand before I could bend down and rescue it. I was distraught. There were dozens of bottles nearby belonging to other athletes, and I was supremely tempted to take a slug, but I thought that would be cheating. Stumbling towards the exit, I hoped there would be an aid station at the start of the course.

As soon as David caught sight of me, I could see by his expression he was concerned. He knew I was in trouble, and so did I. He told me later I looked hot, red and listless. Hardly the way to start a 10-kilometre run. I wasn't just thirsty, I was sapped of energy and momentum and had a long way to go.

The effect of the dehydration was immediate and painfully obvious. The transition from cycling to running is always hard because your legs must get accustomed to a different kind of motion. But this was different. I was devoid of energy, trying to run on empty – and it felt like I had never ever been on a run before. It was like trying to run through wet sand with boots on.

There was no sign of any water.

I stumbled on for the first two kilometres, willing myself to put one foot in front of the other, hoping I would eventually reach an aid station. Finally, right at the top of the course, I reached the first set of volunteers. I could see them in bright tops and baseball caps, holding out bottles and cups and shouting, 'Water? Gatorade?' Not having a clue what Gatorade was, and remembering the triathlon adage *Don't try anything in a race you haven't tried before*, I gulped down a cup of plain old water. I didn't know that Gatorade was in fact exactly what I needed: an energy drink, full of sugar, would have restored me immediately.

In the heat of the mid afternoon sun, with temperatures now edging towards 30°C, I kept glancing down at my Garmin sports watch, which was showing me exactly how slow I was. I was seriously behind my normal pace – just over five minutes per kilometre. I was struggling to do even six minutes per kilometre.

Like the cycle leg of the race, the run was up and down Columbus Drive, with a loop around the spectacular Buckingham Fountain, with its refreshing-looking cascade of tumbling water. This was three and a half laps, and turned out to be not just 10 kilometres but a leg-sapping 11.5.

By the time I saw Mia, Scarlett, Dad and Mark grouped together and straining to see me, I was thinking about giving up. I barely managed a smile as I passed them at snail's pace. I had also stopped looking at my watch; my pace was just depressing me.

But I did look up, and it was then that I started to notice supporters. Not one, not two, but dozens of them all along the route, calling my name and offering brilliant words of encouragement. 'Go on, Louise!' 'You can do it!' 'Head up!' 'Keep smiling!' With every word and golden nugget of advice pushing me on, I limped from one group to another with just enough encouragement to run the next few metres.

By the time I saw my family again, my speed wasn't up, but I had knuckled down. Steely determination had set in, and however painful it was, I knew that I couldn't let down my family, the supporters on the route or the *BBC Breakfast* viewers. I replayed all those tweets of encouragement in my head, and felt shots of willpower every time someone shouted my name. Two and a half laps done and with another lap to go, I was still going slowly but moving forward, and I started to beg people to stay for my last lap. Each group of supporters was like a tiny island of hope in a sea of hot tarmac. As long as they were still there, I could set my sights on them, pass them and then drag myself to the next group – and so on, all the way round the course.

On my final lap, I remember clearly one fellow triathlete, whom I had passed five times, shouting: 'Right, next time it's the finishing straight. When you get there, you are going to take a flag. When you hit the blue carpet, you are going to smile. And then you are going to look up and sprint to the finish line.' I didn't know her then, but Sam Gardiner is now a firm triathlon friend of mine.

After 2 long hours and 36 minutes, buoyed by the incredible support on the course, I finally made it to the last corner of the run. I grabbed a flag from Mark's hands and, just as instructed, looked up when I caught sight of the finish line and started to sprint and smile.

Even at that last moment, the drama wasn't over. I was so exhausted that I stumbled as the flag tangled around my ankle. Immediately, images of me tumbling over in an exhausted heap flashed through my mind, and I only just saved myself from tripping and falling over the finish line.

I could hardly breathe. Struggling to get air into my lungs, I felt like I was suffocating as the officials shook my hand and put my medal around my neck. Lisa and Brij were filming and asking me questions, and for pretty much the first time in my life, I couldn't speak. Dizzy and nauseous, I put my hands on my knees and my head down until my breathing eventually slowed. Then I hobbled over to a paddling pool filled with cold water and ice, and eased myself in to cool off and bring my body temperature down.

I was exhausted, emotionally and physically, and trying to hold back the tears. I had used all my determination to get over the finish line, and now I was euphoric. Enveloped in a huge hug from my family, I knew that every second of struggle and pain had been worth it. I was also incredibly touched to be greeted by three of my fellow age-groupers: Melanie Clarke, Morag McDowall and Ceri Cook had all passed me and then waited patiently to congratulate me on finishing.

After nearly three hours of struggling in the heat of the midday sun, and just over two years after my first triathlon, I had done what I set out to do. This resident of the *BBC Breakfast* sofa, who had given up competitive sport 30 years before, had represented Great Britain in the World Triathlon Championships. I had dared to try – and I had won my personal battle!

There and then, I celebrated as only triathletes do: with an energy drink and a banana!

CHAPTER 20

FOOD, DRINK AND BONKING

'When it came to race-day, I simply hadn't given myself a chance.'

I bet some of you have turned straight to this chapter because of its racy title! Am I right?

Well, until my nearly disastrous race in Chicago I too would have assumed bonking could only be a good thing. When it comes to triathlon, though, it isn't. Let me explain.

To 'bonk' is a term borrowed from cycling, and describes the feeling you have when your body has essentially run out of fuel. Runners, especially marathon runners, would describe it as 'hitting the wall'. Either way, it hurts.

It can happen to anyone, but is more likely after about 90 minutes of moderate to vigorous exercise. Once you have been expending energy for that period, your muscles will have burned all the glucose your body can store in the form of glycogen. If you continue to exercise without replenishing those stores with carbohydrate to produce more blood glucose, your body will start shutting down your muscles, in order to protect your brain.

The medical term for this is hypoglycaemia, and when it happens, it is a horrible and scary feeling. You physically can't make your muscles work because they don't have the fuel to do so.

The problem, in basic terms, is this: to race long distances, you need to eat while you are racing.

An Olympic distance triathlon will take more than 90 minutes for an amateur athlete like me to complete, so fuel can become a big issue – and frequently does. I am by no means alone in making mistakes with hydration and nutrition and then messing up a race. Even top Olympic triathletes can get it wrong, with one particularly notable example.

I am sure you will remember seeing the extraordinary sight of Alistair Brownlee catching, scooping up and dragging his brother Jonathan, who was wobbling, dazed and confused in the heat of the Mexican sun in the Grand Final of the World Championship Triathlon in Cozumel in 2016. The sight of them running together, Jonny's arm slung around Alistair's shoulder for support, and that final moment when Alistair pushed his exhausted younger brother over the finish line, made headlines around the world.

I still recall watching with a mixture of horror and admiration. Horror, because it was quite clear that Jonny was in serious trouble, delirious, with no sense of direction and no control over his legs. Admiration, because of the speed of Alistair's reaction, and that he had both the strength and the presence of mind to grab him, hold him up and get him across the finish line and into the hands of the paramedics.

I have talked to them about that day and where it all went wrong, and this is what they told me. Let's start with Jonny:

'The race was in Mexico and it was very, very hot. If I had won that race I would have become world champion, which would have capped off a very good year. It was all going perfectly well. The swim and bike had all gone well. The guy who I had to beat, the Spanish guy [Mario Mola], was safely in the second pack. It was all going perfect, and then with about a kilometre to go, I thought this is fine, I am going to be world champion, I am going to finish the year off great. I can go home back to Leeds and enjoy myself.

'Then it all went wrong. In the space of about two minutes I went from feeling great to not remembering anything. I only have two memories in the final few minutes. The first memory is Alistair grabbing hold of me and trying to pull me, shouting some very nasty words at me. I was thinking at the time, *Just leave me alone, please leave me alone.* Then the next memory was about half a metre from the finish line, Alistair throwing me across it, and I can't remember anything else.'

Alistair takes up the story:

'I came around the corner, and there he was, swaying in front of me. My first thought when I saw him was, *What an idiot!* This was obviously going to happen, it was hot, he could have won this race so much more easily. My second thought was – and this all happened in a split second – *I must get him to the finish line.* I have been in that position before with heat exhaustion, it's not very nice. I knew I needed to get him some medical attention and get him sorted. So, I ended up kind of dragging him, kind of pulling him down the finish line as quickly as I could. At some point, I thought, *Wait a minute, if he can still get across the finish line in second, he might still win the world title here.* So, at that point I started looking behind me, to see if there was anyone chasing from behind, and I got to the finish line and made sure he got across ahead of me.'

That was the making of one of the most emotional and inspiring moments in sport. Who can forget the television pictures of the two brothers staggering along, Alistair physically dragging Jonny to the finish and sacrificing his own race as he pushed him over the line? What a truly astonishing display of brotherly love!

Jonny had succumbed to heat exhaustion, which can be life-threatening. Alistair explains:

'Heat exhaustion is really dangerous. We have both had it a couple of times, it can happen in quite mild conditions. It is basically when your core temperature gets so hot your body must prioritise your blood going to your lungs and your heart. Everything else starts shutting down. It can be nasty – about 10 per cent fatality if it's not treated quickly. If you are, you tend to come around quite slowly over the next hour, as you are filled with fluids, with lots of ice all over you.'

From a sporting point of view, what Alistair did – and the sacrifice he made – was nothing short of heroic. From a medical perspective, it was the best thing possible. He delivered Jonny straight into the hands of the first aiders, who started to treat him immediately. Within seconds of him landing face down on the blue carpet, water was being poured on his neck and head to cool him down. In hospital, he was put on a drip and recovered quickly: in a few hours, he was tweeting thanks to his older brother, and able to phone his parents to let them know he was OK. After the race, Jonny said that he had been cooling himself down with water during the run by pouring it all over his head, but admitted that he probably hadn't been drinking enough. In the humidity, which makes sweating difficult, this meant that his core body temperature had risen to dangerous levels. Even elite athletes sometimes get it wrong.

My problems in Chicago were a bit more straightforward. In retrospect, they could easily have been prevented. Ceri Cook, who is a Senior Lecturer in Sports Nutrition and Exercise Physiology at the University of Chester and competed alongside me in my age group, said she could see right from the start that I was going to be in trouble.

'I looked at your bike and saw the three jelly sweets, and thought, *That is not going to be enough. You need proper sports energy gels, not sweets.* In an Olympic distance triathlon, when you are going to be on the course for over 90 minutes, you need to fuel properly on the bike to get through the run. In Sprint distance, it is not such an issue, because you are not going to be depleting your body's limited stores of glycogen.'

Even in a race in the UK, I would have been pushing at the limits with only that small amount of food to fuel me. The hot and humid temperatures in Chicago, though, meant that I needed even more food than usual. Ceri later explained to me: 'In the heat, you need even more carbohydrates.'

When it came to race-day, I simply hadn't given myself a chance.

'If you haven't fuelled properly, if you have run out of carbohydrate because the event is over 90 minutes, your body starts using fat oxidisation rather than glycogen stores, which doesn't work so efficiently. You have to slow down, you can't keep going at a high-intensity pace. You feel like you are running through treacle, or sand, or in water; you physically can't speed up.'

Ceri's description of what happens to your body when you have run out of fuel is spot on. What she describes is exactly how I felt in Chicago. Try as I might, there was simply nothing I could do to speed up.

I could have so easily fixed it. All I needed to have done was take an extra gel on the bike, have a carbohydrate drink plus the right amount of water, or gulp down a cup of Gatorade. Then my race would have been a totally different experience. I am not sure I could have run much faster, but I imagine it would have felt a whole lot easier.

And that is the beauty of triathlon: the more you race, the more you know and the better you get. It was only my third Olympic distance race, I had never competed in high temperatures before, and I had no conception of the importance of food and drink. I learned so much from the experience, and have now successfully competed in much longer races, without any sign of a bonk. Best of all, I enjoy those moments sitting on the bike and having something to eat.

As for the triathlon adage *'Don't try anything in a race you haven't tried before'*, desperate times call for desperate measures. Even seasoned competitor Ceri agrees: if you don't think you can feel much worse than you do already, have a cup of whatever the volunteers are offering you!

You just might start to feel a little better.

CHAPTER 21

DON'T GIVE UP.
KEEP TRYING

'The fear that I would have to turn my back on something that I loved challenged me in a host of different and positive ways.'

I can't count the number of times that injury features in our sports bulletins on *BBC Breakfast.* I remember so many of the stories vividly, whether it is David Beckham breaking a metatarsal in his foot; Andy Murray having surgery to sort out his lingering back injury; Rory McIlroy rupturing a ligament playing football with friends; or England hockey captain Kate Walsh fracturing her jaw during the 2012 Olympics. Injury seems to be an integral part of sport.

Nor is this true just at elite level. If you speak to any triathlete, and ask them how training is going, they will normally start the conversation with, 'Well, I have been injured . . .' Then they tell you what they have done and how it affects their training. It can be anything from a fall or crash and breaking something to the much more common sore knees, ankles or – which seems to be the most popular for a triathlete – problems with the Achilles tendon. It seems to me that unless you are superhuman, being injured just goes with the territory. Coping with it, both physically and psychologically, is what makes the difference.

I have had an on and off struggle with injury for years. Now, after lots of advice, help and physiotherapy, I hope I am finally finding the underlying cause and am on my way to solving it. Or, if not solving it, working round it, like so many other people do.

I thought that my problems started with that training for the Great North Run over 10 years ago. Running beside Mia on her bicycle, I tripped over my own feet and twisted my ankle. At the time, it was agony, and I had to hobble back home holding on to her shoulder. Subsequently my whole foot went black and blue. I couldn't put much weight on it, but I presumed I had just bruised it badly. I didn't go to the doctor. I simply stopped running and hoped that it would get better.

It did, but not entirely. About six years later, when the pain went all the way from my foot to my hip, an MRI scan showed that I had in fact broken a little bone in my foot, a metatarsal. I should have spent weeks wearing a protective boot. I naturally assumed that this was where my injury problems began, but I have now realised that the problems go back much further than that.

Matters came to a head as I was training for the European Triathlon Championships in 2016. The British Triathlon system of roll-down places for the Great Britain team meant that I had qualified for Lisbon thanks to my finish time in the Deva Triathlon the previous year. At the time I hadn't even thought about the Euros. I really did think that my international triathlon career would be a one-year wonder. After my experience at the World Championships, though, I had been bitten by the international triathlon bug. Once I knew I had qualified, I was determined to go.

As I trained for the European Championships, I was also training for the New York City Marathon, which I was due to run for *BBC Children in Need* in November that year.

About eight weeks before the European Championships in Lisbon, I did a hard hill session on one of my planned runs – running as fast as I could for one minute up a sharp incline, walking back down again, then repeating eight times. At the time, everything felt fine. More than fine, in fact. I had just taken a break from training for about a week, because I had been suffering from a cold, and to be back out exercising felt great.

That night, I noticed something was wrong: my right knee was swollen to double the size of my left knee. I was a little worried but assumed that if I left it, it would just return to normal. By the morning, it hadn't. Not only was it still swollen, it was also very sore, hurting every time I bent it or tried to walk. I did all the things I thought I should do – put an ice pack on it, took some ibuprofen, and sat with my leg up – and waited for the problem to go away. It didn't.

Concerned, I saw my usual physiotherapist, Gary Bissell at ProPhysio in Chester, who can normally fix anything. On this occasion, though, he told me I needed to go to a doctor. Without an investigation to find out what was wrong, I was in danger of doing long-term damage. I was gutted. I was on the countdown to the European Championships, and my only option now, until I found out what was wrong, was to stop running entirely.

I saw a knee specialist and duly had an MRI scan. The result? Bad news: Patellofemoral trochlear osteochondral defect. Taken aback by the extraordinary name, I asked: 'What on earth is that?'

In simple, non-medical terms, I had a hole in the back of my kneecap. I could see it quite clearly on the scan – it was about the size of a pea. The most likely cause was the pounding on the hill run: it had irritated the area around the damage, causing the inflammation that in turn caused the pain. The worst thing about this was that there was no quick fix. The inflammation might take weeks to go down, if it went down at all, and any running or cycling was likely to aggravate it. All my training for the European Championships, except for swimming, would have to go on hold.

As for my other commitment, training for the New York City Marathon, the consultant was clear about that, too: preparing for a marathon was out of the question. I wouldn't be able to run the long distances required. I was disappointed and very frustrated. I had been training hard for months, and just as I was starting to feel more confident and comfortable, I was going to have to stop.

What about the Euros? I was in a real dilemma: what was I going to do? Was I going to pull out, or give it a go? For me, this was a one-off opportunity. I still wanted to be part of the event, even if that did mean hobbling my way round the course. You can imagine what choice I made. I was determined to race and deal with the consequences afterwards. Continuing to train, I concentrated on swimming and a bit of cycling, but massively reducing the number of miles I ran.

I arrived at the Euros and met up again with the many triathlon friends I had made at the World Championships. It was fantastic to spend a couple of days preparing for the race with Mo McDowall, Ceri Cook and Melanie Clarke, the three women who had waited for me at the finish line of that long, hard race in Chicago. It was good to see them all again and to recce the swim, bike and run course with them.

My knee was still swollen and painful, and the other knee was hurting too, but it wasn't going to stop me competing. Mel, who is a physio, came to the rescue. She strapped both knees up with kinesiology tape, a thin, elastic tape used for therapeutic purposes to treat sports injuries. With a pattern etched in black, it made me look like a warrior with a set of tattoos from my calf, over my knee and halfway up my thigh. I looked and felt much more powerful and strong.

The injury, and the fact that I had hardly been running at all, would make this a challenging race, but the day dawned with a beautiful clear sky. The temperature was warm but not worryingly hot. We swam the 1,500 metres in clear water out and back towards the Lisbon Oceanarium, the largest indoor aquarium in Europe. In the sunshine it became a bright white, shining beacon, so we could easily see where we were heading through the waves.

The bike ride was a 40-kilometre double loop on a closed dual carriageway with stunning views of the River Tagus. We had been warned that there was a hill at the furthest point, but everyone said it was nothing to worry about. They were wrong! It felt like I was going backwards as I struggled to pedal up the 3-kilometre incline and was passed by 20 or so stronger age-groupers. The effort paid off, though, and on the way back I had to hold both the handlebars and my nerve as I reached astonishing speeds downhill of 67 kilometres per hour.

The physio tape on my knees seemed to do the trick on the run. After the exertion on the bike, I did feel like I was running in sand rather than on smooth tarmac, but once again the British supporters were out in force, and I was buoyed up by their exuberance. The atmosphere was brilliant, and I finished the 10-kilometre run in 54.19 – far off my own personal best, but nearly 11 minutes faster than the same distance in Chicago. I loved the whole experience, and I was pleased not to be the last in the Great Britain team.

I went home the proud owner of another International medal, content at the time to believe that I had competed in both a World and European Championship and could now retire, scrunching up my tri suit for ever.

The opposite happened. I came back even more enamoured by the sport. The only sticking point was my problem with my knee. To continue, I would need a long-term solution.

Later that summer, I finally took the advice that Claire had been giving me for months. I made an appointment with a specialist sports physio and chiropractor, Leigh Halfteck, who had helped her with a long-term injury. Specialising in how the nervous system works, he does not treat an injury so much as identify the underlying weakness causing it. In an ideal world, that allows a patient to return to sport not just fixed but as a stronger athlete, one who is less likely to get injured again.

As well as working with sporting giants like Sir Chris Hoy, Leigh had previously been Lead Physiotherapist for the Team GB Taekwondo team, including at the London Olympics. If he could look after people who got kicked for a living, he could certainly look after me.

When I saw Leigh, he asked me lots of questions about injuries or medical issues that I had, going right back to childhood. Apart from my metatarsal I have never broken a bone or bumped my head, but I have had an impressive history of abdominal surgery, including three emergency operations.

The first was when I was about 18 months old and living in Hong Kong. My mum and dad had taken me on holiday to Singapore. One night, they put me to bed as a happy, smiley baby, but when they came to check on me a couple of hours later they had a horrific shock. I was lying listless in a pool of blood, which had soaked through the mattress of my cot. I was rushed to the nearest hospital, where a surgeon took one look at me and diagnosed intussusception, a condition that needed immediate surgery.

Put simply, intussusception is a twisted gut. One part of the intestine telescopes into another, and if left untreated the condition can be life-threatening: I would have died within hours. The surgeon's incisive and quick thinking saved my life, leaving me with what is now a 10-centimetre vertical scar on my stomach.

That was Round One of emergency surgery.

Round Two was 30 years later, and I will spare you too many details. My daughter Mia was born by an emergency caesarean section after midwives realised at the last minute that she was in the breech position – coming into the world bottom rather than head first. Her emergency exit resulted in Scar No. 2.

Round Three was more alarming.

A week after Mia was born, racked with excruciating stomach pain and an extremely high temperature of 41°C, I was readmitted to hospital. None of the doctors could work out what was wrong with me, and two days later my appendix burst, though they only realised this had happened after they opened me up to investigate.

That emergency surgery left me with three additional scars, and once again saved my life.

It is only thanks to modern medicine, and the doctors and nurses involved in every operation, that I am still here to tell the tale. The only downside is that my stomach looks like Spaghetti Junction, a criss-cross of scars. I am grateful for and proud of those scars: without them, I wouldn't be here.

For Leigh, though, the scars were the problem. He thought that the various incisions had cut my nerves, tissue and muscles so many times that the scar tissue was affecting the way I moved my legs. By constricting my stomach muscles, they made it hard for me to run, which was damaging my knees. Even my internal organs, he believed, were probably now in the wrong place.

This was a revelation to me. For all those years struggling, I had been fighting against the scars. Leigh set me a series of exercises to do at home, specifically designed to strengthen the weaknesses that I had been working around for decades.

The change was almost immediate: within a few weeks my knee stopped swelling and I was pain-free. For the first time in months, I could get up in the morning without hobbling. Running still wasn't my favourite sport, but instead of being hunched up like a hermit crab in a borrowed shell, I began to feel that I was running free – upright and, possibly, a little faster.

The relief was immense.

My injuries obviously pale into insignificance compared to those of so many other people, but I had nonetheless found dealing with them debilitating, frustrating and sometimes downright depressing.

In the run-up to the Euros, trying to cope with the pain had worn me down. Sometimes I couldn't sleep or I woke up in the night, or putting my foot in the wrong place suddenly caught me out. I tend to be tired anyway from waking up in the early hours to go to work, but the constant discomfort consumed me. Just as frustrating was the thought that if I couldn't race, all those hours of hard training during the long winter months, and the incremental improvements I had made, would be for nothing.

What made me the most anxious, though, was the fear that my knee injury might mean giving up triathlon altogether. Might mean turning my back on something that I loved and which challenged me in a host of different and positive ways, making me feel strong, fit and focused.

So you can imagine my feelings when Leigh got me back running again. I had to start right back with the basics, running for just a minute at a time and then walking, and very slowly building it up from there; but to know that I would be able to continue with my sport was empowering. I was still far from being back to running 10 kilometres, and even further still from being able to train for, let alone finish a marathon – but at least I was back running.

The lesson I take from this episode is simple: with injuries, you have to keep looking for a solution. If you don't find one, try to find a way through it, or a way round it. Tenacity, resilience and a great physio can get you through.

CHAPTER 22

TOO LATE TO BACK OUT

'I hate running and I only do it because I have to, and I only run a maximum of 10 kilometres.'

The first thing to say about my experience running a marathon is this: I would not recommend it to anyone. It is painful to do – and when you haven't trained properly, dangerous – but it is also one of the most life-affirming things I have ever done.

As you know from reading this far, I *love* triathlons but I really don't like running. In fact, I would go so far as to say that I hate running. A marathon was not something I had ever dreamed of doing, and I was adamant that I would never volunteer to do one either, even under duress. It can be infuriating when people say: 'Never say never', but I was *never* going to attempt to run a marathon.

So, in November 2015, when I had a call from Hiten Vora, the enthusiastic personal assistant to Radio 2's Chris Evans, I found myself in a dilemma. I always love Hiten's calls because they invariably involve some madcap but brilliant idea. The call went along these lines:

'Hey, Lou, we know you are a runner with all your triathlon and everything. Well, we are going to auction a hugely exciting marathon package on Radio 2 to raise money for *Children in Need* and we need your help.'

I stopped him right there and said: 'Hold on, Hiten, I hate running and I only do it because I have to, and I only run a maximum of 10 kilometres.'

He ignored me and carried on. 'The thing is, the package is going to include a place in the London Marathon, the Windsor Half Marathon and the New York City Marathon. Paula Radcliffe is going to help with the training, and when you all finish she will take everyone out for a celebratory dinner in New York. Chris is going to do London and Windsor, but this is the reason why I am calling: he can't do New York. We would love it if you would do it on his behalf.'

As I said, I thought I was *never* going to run a marathon, but what do you do when you get a call like that? Say: 'Sorry, I can't. I am too busy/just can't be bothered/might be washing my hair'?

Chris's listeners are incredibly generous and raise staggering amounts of money for *Children in Need*, so if I were to help in any way I would just have to get over my marathon phobia and give it a go.

After a couple of days of thinking, I told Hiten I would try, and so, in the run-up to *Children in Need* in November, when the magnificent marathon package was auctioned on BBC Radio 2, my name was included as part of the experience. Once I had been mentioned to the millions of listeners, it was too late to back out.

Just as I thought, there was a bidding frenzy for the marathon prize. By the end of the auction, the successful bidders had raised £282,229 for the running package alone – an astounding amount of money. There really was no way of turning back.

Over the last few years, I have visited several of the charities supported by *Children in Need*. I had always wanted to see where the money is spent, and I am lucky enough to have met some of the children it has helped and to have spoken to their parents, who have all told me about the huge difference the money has made to their lives. So, I was determined to get a grip and to start putting in those training miles. I knew the training was going to be both time-consuming and tough, and to make it more challenging I also wanted to continue my triathlon training because there was still a chance of qualifying for a place in the European Championships in Lisbon in May 2016.

The training did not go as planned, and I was devastated.

Just as I was getting better at running and coping with longer distances, I was injured, as you know from the previous chapter. Having been told by the consultant that there was no way I could train for a marathon, I rang the Radio 2 team with a heavy heart. My marathon attempt was over before it had even begun. All was not lost, though: after some discussion, they told me they would still like me to go and support the rest of the team on their journey to New York.

After a summer of hardly doing any running at all, my knee stopped hurting. Inevitably, thoughts about the New York City Marathon returned to haunt me. I was going to be travelling there anyway, so was there any way I could possibly run? Could I perhaps attempt to walk it? Was I absolutely bananas to even think about it?

With about six weeks to go, I asked both my physio, Leigh, and coach, Claire, if perhaps they thought I could run or walk it? They came back in unison: no way! Even walking it would be risky. I hadn't done the training and I was more than likely to injure myself again, possibly with long-term consequences.

They had almost persuaded me to abandon the idea. Then, the week before I was due to go to New York, *Breakfast* asked me to film an interview with a young girl, which would be shown for *Children in Need* week.

When she was aged 11, her father was diagnosed with cancer and died shortly afterwards, leaving mother and child to face life without him. Just three years later, the two of them were faced with the devastating news that her mum also had terminal cancer. The girl was just 15 and in her GCSE year at the time of her mother's death.

Through all those tough years, she had been to see a grief counsellor for one hour a week, every week. That session was funded by donations to *Children in Need*. We met at the hospice where both her parents had spent time before they died, and she talked to me eloquently about her experiences of grief, and about how much the weekly counselling had helped her open up and reach out during those dark days when she didn't think she could cope. This strong and quietly determined young woman, who has been helped on her way in life by other people's generosity, made a lasting impression on me.

Inspired by her story, I had a moment of clarity, and on the day before flying to New York I packed my trainers. The very least I could do, on behalf of all those who give money to *Children in Need*, and those who have been helped by the charity, was to start the marathon and see what happened.

The only person I told about my madcap plan was David. During those months of injury, he too had thought it was exactly what I should do. We didn't tell anyone else – not Mia, not Scarlett, not Mum or Dad, and certainly not my coach, Claire!

CHAPTER 23

HOW NOT TO RUN A MARATHON

'In life, you don't need things, you need experiences.'

Jill Douglas, the world's chattiest running companion

It was madness even to contemplate starting.

The last time I had run 10 kilometres was six months previously in May, at Lisbon for the European Championships. Since then, my injured knee meant that the furthest I had run was about three and a half miles – and even that had only been once.

So, when the day of departure arrived and I met up with the *BBC Children in Need* team of runners at Heathrow on our way to New York, I was quite clear that I had decided only to start the marathon. I would not attempt to finish it – because that would be complete lunacy.

When I made my plan, what I didn't appreciate was that starting but not finishing is easier said than done.

Wherever I decided to leave the marathon, I would most likely end up miles from the finish, and it might be difficult to get back either to the finish or to where we were staying. While all the other *Children in Need* marathoners prepared for the race, my main priority was to choose an easy and safe place to leave, and decide whether I would take the subway or walk back.

What I needed was local knowledge.

Luckily, my friend Matt Ford lives in New York with his wife, Katrina, affectionately known as Treens. She has been a friend since we were at the University of St Andrews together. Matt had successfully run the race twice, and knew the city inside out.

Over a glass of wine and some carb-loading pasta in a wonderful noisy Italian restaurant, we had a long discussion about strategy. He told me there were only two places I could quit running and get back to Manhattan easily. One was at about Mile 8 in Brooklyn, where I could walk a couple of blocks, then catch the subway. The other was at Mile 16, just after the course crossed over the Queensboro Bridge, into Manhattan and on to First Avenue.

If I managed to get that far – and it was a big if – I could hobble back up 59th Street to Central Park. Matt was adamant that I should not attempt to run any further than that, and vividly described the long miles up First Avenue into the Bronx, through Harlem and back up the hill to Central Park as some of the toughest, most soul-destroying running he had done in his life.

Mile 8? That would be pushing it, but I figured that I could walk my way there. As for Mile 16, that sounded ridiculous, even after a glass of red wine!

Waking in the early hours of marathon day, excited about the challenges ahead, and running in the dark to find our bus to take us to the start, I had a clear plan: get to Mile 8, then see how I was doing. If, by some miracle, I was OK, I would push on to Mile 16, where I would meet David and we would then walk back to the hotel. Either of the options was way beyond my comfort zone. I wasn't fit to run 10 kilometres, let alone 26.2 miles.

The team running that day was made up of some very serious runners. There was Vassos Alexander, Radio 2's sports presenter and a fabulously fast long-distance runner. There were Ewan and Jane from Edinburgh. Jane had taken up running only when she was 50, but 26.2 miles would be a relaxed day out for the pair of them; they specialised in ultramarathons and fell running. There were Mark and Wendy from Torquay. Mark had run for years, but Wendy was a new runner: when Mark had bought them a running machine only a year before the marathon, she could complete no more than a mile. There was Jules, another ultrarunner, who had been signed up by his wife for the marathon package as a surprise Christmas present and who had already won a 200-mile race in Arctic conditions – he had been the only person to complete the course. There were also two very experienced veteran runners on board, Liam and Carl, and a new runner, 61-year-old Jill Douglas.

Jill is an amazing lady, whose decision to take up running at age 60 came on the spur of the moment, as she was listening to the *Chris Evans Breakfast Show*. She had gone to spend all her savings on a new car. The dealer in the showroom was so rude to her that she had turned on her heel and driven home in her own car, leaving her bank account intact, listening to the *Children in Need* auction on Radio 2.

Inspired by the idea of the marathon auction, and the money being pledged, Jill made a fateful call to the radio station and started bidding. Only a few minutes later she had donated her entire savings to charity and signed herself up to both the London and New York City marathons. 'The next morning I woke up and thought, I have just blown all my savings! But it is such a worthy cause, I am still fit and active enough to be able to run a marathon, and who needs another car? You don't need more stuff when you get to a certain age.'

It was an extraordinary act of generosity. Jill had never run before, and like me, she didn't much enjoy it. Even so, she set about dedicating her year to learning to love it, starting with a fitness class three days a week and progressing to, in her words, 'shuffling' around Virginia Water in Windsor Great Park.

With such an attitude, I knew that of all the people in the *Children in Need* team, I wanted to run with her.

At sunrise, packed on to the steamy bus whisking us out to the start on Staten Island, we were all talking nineteen to the dozen about our plans, imagining which would be the toughest bits, and whether we would ever run marathons again.

I sat next to Jill, and asked if she would be happy to let me run with her. I knew that we would be the slowest runners of our group, so my hope was that we could stick together, keep each other company and chat through the pain.

Security was very tight as we joined thousands of other runners pressed together ahead of the check-in, watched closely by intimidating NYPD officers in dark sunglasses and sleek black rifles slung over their shoulders. It was chilly, but the atmosphere was fizzing with anticipation. In the long queues, runners wrapped up in warm clothes chatted to each other as we gently jostled our way through the police screening. I was delighted when I bumped into some *BBC Breakfast* fans who were also running.

Because the members of our team were all planning to run at a varying pace, we had been put into different waves. The speedy ones – Vassos, Jules, Liam, Carl and Mark – left first, and the rest of us had an hour or so to hang about and wait.

For once in my life, I wasn't at all nervous, just enjoying being part of the crowd and watching everyone getting ready: eating, drinking, resting, stretching. I realised I didn't have my name on my running top and managed to find a black felt-tip sharpie so Jill could write 'Louise, UK' in big letters on my chest. I was hoping that the crowd shouting my name might help motivate me.

At 10 a.m. on the dot, I jumped in fright at the sound of a loud boom. It was the cannon blasting for the first wave to start.

The event was incredibly well organised. Each wave of runners was sorted by estimated finishing time, and had a clearly marked starting pen. With half an hour or so to go before we were due to start, Ewan, Jane, Jill and I made our way towards the pens. We were meant to be in different ones, but at Jill's encouragement we managed to wriggle our way into one pen to wait together. It was much warmer than I had expected, the autumn sunshine heating up our backs as we shuffled from foot to foot, and everyone started to shed layers of clothing into large donation bins.

At 10.40 a.m. exactly, we were released from the pens and started the slow walk towards the Verrazano-Narrows Bridge, which connects Staten Island to Brooklyn. It is an impressive double-decker suspension bridge over a large expanse of water. Legend has it that runners on the top level, nervous and having missed the last loo stop, pee over the edge, so those on the bottom row get covered in urine. A disgusting thought, especially as we were due to run on the lower deck. My fellow runners assured me that it was just a marathon legend – and I'm delighted to confirm to you that was indeed the case.

The start was so different to my experiences of triathlon, where everyone is fidgeting nervously and revved up, ready to race. It was surprisingly calm, and even a little emotional as we listened to a glorious rendition of 'God Bless America' resounding through the sound system.

As the gun boomed again to herald our start, Jill and I set off together, relaxed and excited about the road ahead. Immediately, the chatter from the runners surrounding us stopped, and an eerie silence washed over us as we jogged slowly over the bridge. I looked over to our left and was very touched to see a fireboat pumping plumes of foaming water into the air in a fantastic display of support.

I knew that I was going to have to start slowly if I was going to have a chance of going any distance at all, and I tried not to get carried away by the river of runners. The first kilometre over the bridge was dominated by a silent jostling, as everyone tried to find their happy pace. But as we left the Verrazano-Narrows Bridge and ran through Dyker Heights, the atmosphere changed. Instead of running in silence, we were greeted by rousing raucous crowds waving and cheering encouragement. Seeing my name scrawled on my T-shirt, they yelled: 'Go Louise', 'You got this, Louise', 'Go on, Louise, you got this.' If they had only known how unprepared I was; I hadn't got it at all!

For the first few miles, Jill and I seemed to be trotting along surprisingly easily, and to my amazement the miles started to tick by steadily. There was no hint of pain in my knee, and when I looked at my watch I could see that we were doing really well. In fact, if anything, we were moving a little too fast. Never in my life had I run as happily, but we were going to have to keep it nice and steady to go the distance, so I kept saying to Jill, 'Let's slow down.'

By Mile 6, I was feeling amazing, and for the first time began to think I might not stop at Mile 8.

We had been trotting on at such a pace that we missed my husband, David, on a bend in Bay Ridge. Then, as we made our way up Boerum Hill in Brooklyn, he shouted at us from the back of the crowd and squeezed his way through to join us. I didn't even break my pace, and he ran along beside us while we talked animatedly about how much fun we were having, and I told him that I was going to crack on.

The only problem I had was that I was hungry already. Once again, I had made a massive miscalculation. Assuming I was going to give up, I hadn't bothered to take any food or gels with me. My experience at the World Championships in Chicago was playing on my mind, but I thought I had a solution. As we moved away from David and up the hill, I shouted: 'See you at 16, and please can you get me a Snickers bar?' At the same time, I could hear the voice of my coach, Claire, in my head: *You are running a marathon on a Snickers bar? That's crazy!*

From Brooklyn onwards, the noise and support from the crowds and bands playing on the side of the roads was so intense it was almost overwhelming.

We kept on running, running, running. The sheer enthusiasm from the crowds pushed us further and further on our mad endeavour. Then, at Mile 10 in Williamsburg, we heard a loud shout: 'Jill! Jill!' For the first time, my brilliant running partner left my side and rushed across the road into the arms of her two grown-up sons, Jonathan and Mark. They gave us both huge hugs, Jill shed a tear, and then they sent us back on our way. For Jill, after years of cheering on her sons from the sidelines, it was a wonderful role reversal: 'It was so uplifting to see them there, so nice to see their familiar faces, willing me to do it. I wouldn't give up because I didn't want to let them down, you don't want to feel that you have failed.'

Buoyed by their enthusiasm, we were in great spirits and still going strong until the road spiralled up a steep ramp to the brutally intimidating Queensboro Bridge. This steel cantilevered structure towers over the East River, using Roosevelt Island like a stepping stone from Queens into Manhattan.

The moment we stepped on to the bridge, an icy crosswind blasted us, chilling us to the bone. It was also eerily quiet. No spectators were allowed up there with us, and it felt as if a malevolent force had flicked a switch and turned off the sound of the crowd. Along the mile-long span of the bridge, runners were breaking down and collapsing. One young girl was horrified, with tears streaming down her face. I put my arm around her and tried to encourage her, but she said she was too upset to go on. Gently we persuaded her, and the last we saw of her she was speeding ahead of us on to First Avenue.

The arrival of the marathon from Queens into Manhattan is fabled among long-distance runners. And, just as I had been told, I could hear the roar of the crowd several minutes before I could see them.

At Mile 16, we rounded the corner of 59th Street and First Avenue and were met by hundreds of smiling faces, 20 feet deep, lining both sides of the road.

Unbelievably, among all those people, my friends Treens and Matt were shouting so loudly I could hear them: 'Lou, Lou, here is your Snickers bar!' And there they were, holding out the bar for me to grab.

That was where I was meant to stop. Get out, climb over the barrier, and leave.

It didn't happen.

I am not sure, even now, at what point I decided to finish the marathon. Somewhere on those long miles, my subconscious had decided that I would carry on if we were still together at Mile 16. Well, there we were, still running elbow to elbow. There didn't seem to be a choice: having run so far, stopping would let both Jill and myself down.

Afterwards she told me, 'I know you didn't intend to do the whole thing, but once you start it is hard to bottle out. You just keep going, and with someone else you feel a bit more courageous, a bit more daring, a bit bolder. We just kept each other going, and it is great to run with somebody like that.'

The miles ahead might be tough – but we both knew they were not as numerous as the miles behind us.

I ran past the rosestone Church of St. John Nepomucene, dwarfed by the skyscrapers beside it, and saw David waiting for me. This was the exact point where I had said I would leave. Instead, I gave him a huge hug and told him I was going to carry on. He had already guessed I would; he knows me much better than I know myself.

By then, Jill and I were suffering, and had adopted a run–walk strategy – possibly better described as a walk–shamble strategy. Each aid station, manned by dozens of volunteers in bright green ponchos, was like a lifeline pulling us forward. Reaching one at each mile marker meant that we could walk again while grabbing a cup of water or an energy drink. Then about a hundred metres beyond, we would try to run again.

Hard doesn't begin to describe the miles through the Bronx and Harlem. I am not sure I was making much sense by then. Jill had been telling me about what happens when you hit the wall, insisting that it wasn't just a physical breakdown but a mental one as well. I naively assumed that we were going too slowly for that to happen to us – but at Mile 18, Jill went very quiet. I was worried by her change in mood.

By Mile 20, though, she had cheered up and was chatting again. It seemed not to matter that we were now slower and slower. I could only walk the seemingly endless miles up Fifth Avenue. Eventually we turned the corner into Central Park, just as it was beginning to get dark. I was over the moon to see David and Matt and Treens waving madly at us. Treens was overcome, crying as she gave me a restorative hug. I began to think, *Surely, I can do this! I'm nearly there, aren't I?*

Almost in sight of the finish, at Mile 24, screeching agony overtook me. Every nerve, tendon, ligament and muscle was screaming with shooting pain. Even my face was hurting. I couldn't bear to put one foot in front of the other. All I wanted to do was curl up by the side of the road, put my hands over my head and sob like a toddler.

I had hit the wall.

Jill was brilliant. 'Come on, Louise, you have had two children. It cannot be worse than having them.'

It was.

Actually, it was much worse.

Trying to run downhill, I was in excruciating pain. I had lost all sense of purpose and direction. My willpower was gone.

A skinny, tall New Yorker in his late fifties caught up with me, wearing a T-shirt emblazoned with the words 'Cancer survivor' on the back. He told me that this was the fourth time he had run the marathon, this time after receiving treatment for cancer. Now he was clear.

Well, that was more than motivational, it was exactly what I needed to give me a kick in the butt!

By the time I lost sight of him, I had made it to Mile 25, out of the park. All I had to do was stumble through the last stretch up 59th Street, then loop back to catch our first glimpse of the finish ahead of us in the dusk.

The blue banner stretched across the road, with grandstands on either side, looked like an oasis. I have never been happier to see a finishing line in my life. With one last effort, I tried as best I could to at least appear as if I was running. Jill managed a huge triumphant smile as we virtually fell over the line together, side by side, just as we had been every single step of the race.

It had taken us an agonising 5 hours and 50 long minutes. Almost by mistake, I had done it: finished a marathon, achieved the impossible and gone far beyond my expectations. All I wanted to do now was cry.

As it was, I could hardly stay on my feet as one of the thousands of volunteers put a massive silver finishing medal round my neck. I just managed to hold it up and break out an exhausted smile for an official photo. Then, for the first time that day, I was separated from Jill. She had to pick up her bag, and I was directed to a different exit.

It got very dark very quickly, and I started to shiver in the drizzle that was falling.

As I hobbled alongside other finishers in similar states of distress, it began to dawn on me that it was going to be a long way back to the hotel. The exit was halfway up Central Park, which meant the hotel was about 20 blocks away – at least one more mile.

With 50,000 runners all finishing in one place, the organisers had closed most of the surrounding streets to funnel us back safely into the city. There were no taxis, no subways – and, since we hadn't planned where to meet at the finish, there was no wonderful husband to help me or give me a hug. I was facing a painful stumble home.

I managed to hold back the tears until the moment I was enveloped in a fluffy blue poncho by a volunteer. She did it up for me with such a sweet smile that she set me off, and the tears started tumbling down my cheeks. I cry very seldom, but now the floodgates opened and I just couldn't stop. I could hardly breathe for the sobbing, and for the first time in the whole day I was gulping for air. Though surrounded by dozens of equally shattered runners in matching bright blue ponchos, I felt utterly alone. I couldn't talk to anyone. Just put my head down and kept walking, the tears streaming uncontrollably down my face.

Forty minutes later, and after staggering my way miserably through the dark and windy streets of New York, I had just about got the tears under control when I finally reached the bright lights of the hotel lobby. There, waiting to greet me, was none other than marathon runner extraordinaire Paula Radcliffe. Breathtakingly glamorous, she was going to take all of us *Children in Need* runners out for a final celebration dinner.

Allison Curbishley, a former 400-metre runner who had been looking after all of us during the Marathon year, had been texting Paula to try to get her to stop me running. So the sight of me with a medal round my neck was almost as much of a surprise to Paula as it was to me. She bounced over to wrap me up in the most enormous congratulatory hug. That set off the tears again. By the time David came and found me, I was blubbing like a baby.

It only took one beer and a blissfully warm bath to transform the tears into laughter.

I discovered that I wasn't alone in finding it a challenging day. In fact, everyone had found it a very tough race. Vassos felt so ill that he didn't even make it to dinner; he was shivering, white as a sheet and clearly running a temperature. He took himself straight to the airport, missing dinner. Jules had collapsed just a mile from the finish, lying in a star shape on the ground with his whole body in a spasm. After receiving first aid, he managed to haul himself to the finish line, and was able to join us at the celebration dinner.

Jill and I were both hurting, but we had come out of it relatively lightly. Though I was now hobbling and would be stiff for the next few days, I knew from the way I had felt during the race, and immediately afterwards, that I hadn't done myself any long-term damage. Mentally, I was buzzing, with a sense of elation and pride. It was magical and inspiring to have been part of a massive human endeavour. One of 50,000 people, all facing the same challenge.

The support of Jill, the other runners, the New Yorkers lining the route to cheer us, and the glimpses of David, Treens and Matt helped me to the finish line. Helped me realise, too, that I can be more resilient, determined and tenacious than I ever imagined.

I will always remember Jill's words: 'In life, you don't need things, you need experiences.'

I couldn't agree more. That day was life-affirming and it will be with me for ever. After all those years of thinking I don't like running, maybe I do? Perhaps I just need to dare to try some more.

CHAPTER 24

JUGGLING

'I normally run for an hour or so, and whatever has happened at work – good, bad or indifferent – soon becomes a distant memory.'

I won't lie. It isn't always easy juggling a busy family life, presenting *Breakfast* and trying to be a British Triathlon age-group athlete. The truth is, it is hard, it requires effort, determination and sacrifice, and it is sometimes a logistical nightmare. Almost always it is the triathlon training that gets squeezed, but I try my best.

Planning is essential and I always have a training schedule for the week, set by my coach, Claire. It normally consists of at least one or two hour-long swim sessions, a couple of different bike sessions, at least three run sets, and perhaps a strength and conditioning or physio session. She normally plans about eight hours a week and I try to fit it in around home life, my children's school, social arrangements and work.

Claire sets the days she would like me to do things, but I am always swapping them around because my plans are often changing. For example, I might suddenly need to go to London to do an interview after the programme. By the time I have finished presenting, caught the train down, done the interview and caught the train back home again, it is late and that will rule out any exercise, so I will have to try another day.

On the other hand, if I didn't work on *BBC Breakfast* and instead worked 9 to 5, I would struggle to do even half the training I manage. One of the positive things about getting up when most other people are in bed is that my work is normally finished much earlier than everyone else. On a good day, it means I can sneak in some training while Mia and Scarlett are still at school, have it done by the time I pick them up, and then spend time with them.

These days, on a day when I am presenting, my alarm goes off at 3.30 a.m. I really try not to press the snooze button because being woken up twice in the early hours seems to make me feel even more grotty than normal, but I do often succumb to the temptation. I get into work by 5 a.m., an hour before I am on air. By then I will already have a good idea of the guests we have and the stories we are covering. We have a brief editorial meeting to discuss our lead story, highlight any concerns or things to look out for, and then it is time for my most crucial appointment of the day: make-up! That takes about 30 minutes.

After a quick rehearsal of the headlines at about five to six, we are off for three and a quarter hours of live broadcasting to more than six and a half million people. The time seems to fly because there is so much to think about. *What are the headlines? What is coming up next? What am I going to ask? Am I happy with my questions? What was that Carol said about the temperature? Did the director say Camera 4 or 6?*

It is so intense that when we come off air at 9.15 a.m. I go into a sort of post-*Breakfast* dream state; it is almost like I am punch-drunk and am unable to answer a simple question or make a decision. The best way to come around from that is exercise. So, when I get home, I plan to do a swim, bike or run.

Waffle, my Labrador, loves it when it is a running day. As soon as she sees me change out of my presenting clothes and put on my trainers, she knows this is her chance for an adventure. Before I am even out of the house, she runs in circles around me with a sock or a tennis ball in her mouth, whining and increasingly desperate to get going. I normally run for an hour or so, and whatever has happened at work – good, bad, or indifferent – soon becomes a distant memory. On a running day, I don't seem to care much about the weather. Even if it is cold or raining, I still head out; after a few minutes I will warm up anyway. And if I am wet, freezing and covered in mud when I get back home, a long soak in a hot bath will soon cure that.

By contrast, I am a fair-weather cyclist. I hate being out on my bike in the cold or rain, so the only way I can train effectively in the winter is on an indoor bike. I used to train for a couple of hours a week while watching telly or doing homework for *BBC Breakfast* on a static spinning bike – a bit like one of those cycles you see being used in gyms.

I have now graduated to training on a smart turbo trainer, as described on page 62. The advantage of a turbo is that you are riding the same bike that you will be riding when you venture outside on to the road again. In short, you'll be bike fit. I find it a brilliant way of training: it cuts down the faff of getting all my gear ready, and means that in the winter months I am not cycling on slippery roads in the cold, watching out for cars.

Technology has now taken me a step further than that, and I have started gaming on my bike. I never expected to become a gamer at the age of 48, and it has revolutionised my training. I link my turbo trainer to my computer, which measures how fast I am pedalling and how much power I am creating, and then sends the information to Zwift, an online cycling game. That information powers my online cycling avatar – and this is where things get clever. In real time, I can cycle with or against other people from all over the world, in a virtual environment. It is a cyclist's utopia: smooth tarmac, open roads, no cars, no potholes, and no real rain. Plus there's the opportunity for some healthy competition, to drive you on.

My favourite thing to do on Zwift is to join a group ride.

There is one on a Sunday night, which I join as often as possible. It is ostensibly a women's ride, but men join it as well, and we always tease them when they do. Wherever we are in the world, we set off simultaneously for a ride that takes an hour or so. The ride leader sets the pace, and there are normally about 70 of us from different time zones: Japan, New Zealand, Australia and America. We can see each other and send messages to the group, and we try to stick together on the course and help each other up hills and on sprints. Some days I have real trouble keeping up; on others I can be leading from the front. Either way, it is great fun to see our avatars all cycling alongside each other.

Being online also means that I cycle more often – harder, faster and for much longer, too. Apart from competing in a real triathlon, there is nothing quite like coming first in the sprint and my avatar wearing the yellow jersey for a few minutes.

Of course, the best sort of cycling is IRL (In Real Life), as my fellow Zwifters say. For me, that means a warm, sunny summer afternoon, whizzing along a route from Chester across the Burton Marshes, over a boardwalk and towards Little Neston. I pick my way past the fluffy white sheep grazing on the rough grass while drinking in the glorious views of the Welsh hills across the Dee Estuary. It is not often I can fit in one of those bike rides, but it always lifts my spirits.

Fitting in the swimming is always the biggest struggle, almost always a battle of mind over matter. Even as I write this, I should be swimming 3,000 metres!

The thing is, I *love* swimming, but I don't love *going* for a swim. I don't like the practicalities of it – getting wet and getting dry again. I will do almost anything to wriggle my way out of going for a swim, so I have learned to make it virtually impossible not to get in the pool. On a swimming day, to trick my way into it, I take all my kit – goggles, hat, costume, towel, shampoo, etc. – to work, and then drive straight to the pool afterwards so there is absolutely no room for a diversion.

Even that doesn't always work. There are weeks when I take my swimming kit to work every day and then, at the last moment, change my mind and find some lame excuse not to go on that particular day. I try not to feel like a failure, though I know I am letting myself down. I know I would love swimming once I get in, if only I could get over that initial hurdle.

In the summer, I find it much easier. Even though open-water swimming involves wetsuits and colder temperatures, it seems altogether better and more manageable. There are lots of wonderful places to swim where I live in Cheshire – supervised and therefore safe. There is something about the camaraderie of lining up on the water's edge, gingerly splashing my way through the shallows, shivering as I brave the cold and then setting off with conviction to swim a 750-metre circuit alongside lots of other people. I can also never resist the temptation of trying to outpace someone who is slightly faster than me, which adds to the fun.

At the end of a normal week, jostling and juggling the exercise, I usually manage to complete about 90 per cent of the eight hours' training that Claire has set me – so between six and seven hours. Compared to most triathletes I have asked in the British Triathlon team, that's way down the bottom of the scale, but much more would be virtually impossible.

I couldn't begin to do this level of training if I didn't have a huge amount of determination, and that is driven by two distinct types of motivation.

There is what I call the *macro motivation*, by which I mean the reasons why I am embarking on it in the first place. One: it makes me feel fit, strong and happy. Two: training means racing, and I love racing. Three: racing well means I can be in the Great Britain team, which makes me proud and excited.

Without the macro motivation, I couldn't have the *micro motivation*, the drive to make dozens of decisions on an almost daily basis to put on my trainers, get in the pool, or get out on my bike – all of which add together to make it possible for me to be on the start line.

For each of the three disciplines, my micro motivation seems very different.

I love the cycling, whether outside or inside, and I will almost always complete what Claire has set me for the week. Now I am a gamer on Zwift, I will often exceed what she has planned for me.

As for running, technology has the effect of ensuring there is nowhere to hide and no way to pretend I have done things I haven't. The heart rate monitor, sports watch and the power metre on my bike all connect to the Internet and to a system called Training Peaks, where Claire sets my training plan. After every training session, it uploads automatically, and she can see, for example, exactly how far I have run, what pace I ran, and what my heart rate was. This means she can track my progress, and see if I am getting fitter and faster.

Encouraged by the exuberant Waffle and her voracious appetite for exercise, I am happy to run whatever the weather, but I continually cut corners and feel guilty about it. More often than not I will do only 50 minutes instead of the hour that Claire has set me, or only six hill efforts instead of seven. Even on the athletics track I find some silly excuse not to do the last set. There is something about getting to the end of a run that I find psychologically challenging, and frequently I don't quite complete what I am meant to do.

If only my approach to swimming and running were the same as to cycling! Then I would fly along, and smash my way into the team.

There is no doubt that having a coach is important for me; it really helps with the juggling. I know that Claire is an expert, who knows my goals. This gives me confidence: if I follow her directions as best as I can, then the likelihood is that I will achieve what I have set out to do. Having her plan everything also takes an enormous amount of stress out of it. I never have to work out what type of run or bike ride I should do, or worry whether I am optimising my time spent training; I just get on and do it.

Having your own coach is a luxury, there's no doubt about it. Someone who makes me swim, cycle and run is the way I 'treat' myself. Without a coach I would not have been able to achieve what I have in a sport that I love, and in such a short space of time. If you don't want your own coach or the price is too high, there are lots of free, online training programmes, which will take you from the couch to a 5-kilometre run, or help you plan your first sprint triathlon.

My advice would be, don't be overambitious. Choose a plan that you are going to be able to complete. There is nothing more demoralising and demotivating than always struggling to finish the week's exercise sessions. Most triathlon clubs run coaching sessions for swimming, running and cycling, either for free or just a couple of pounds each. The added advantage of a Tri Club session is that you will meet fellow triathletes – and pick up masses of valuable but free advice. In my experience, there is only one thing triathletes love more than training, and that is talking about their sport.

What I can't do, but which I know would be really useful, is have a regular training partner. For me, one working week is invariably different from the next, so I can't guarantee that I will be available to train at a certain time on a certain day. I know that training with someone would help keep me motivated; with a partner for an hour's run, I wouldn't be stopping at 50 minutes. I also find that a good chat along the way is brilliantly distracting. For the time being, though, I still have the wonderful Waffle and very occasionally a reluctant husband!

To answer the original question, 'How do I juggle?', I struggle. Struggle to juggle, but manage to juggle because I have a plan, a heavy dose of motivation and the experience that every time I finish a session I feel better about everything in general – and a little happier about myself.

CHAPTER 25

RELAY: THE BEST WAY

'I made a very quick change out of my smart presenting clothes in the ladies' loo, tied my hair in a ponytail and dashed down to the start.'

You might be under the impression that triathlon is a sport aimed at individuals, but one of my favourite ways to race a triathlon is as part of a relay.

If you have been reading this and are now thinking of trying triathlon out for the first time, relays are a great way to start. You can experience the fun and madness of being part of the race, but with the advantages of only having to compete in your favourite sport or discipline.

Triathlon relays can take all sorts of different forms, and in my experience all are equally enjoyable. In some ways, the more chaotic they are, the more fun they are.

You can do the most conventional form of tri-relay, which is three people in a team, one doing each discipline in sequence, and then passing the timing chip on to each other in transition. Or you can have much bigger teams and longer relays, like the one I took part in for *Sport Relief*, called the Leaderboard Triathlon.

That race took place in the artificial lake at Eton Dorney in Berkshire, which was used as the rowing and canoe sprint venue for the Olympics in London 2012. It was the biggest mass relay I have ever seen – and great fun.

The rules were flexible, but to finish the race, each team of up to six people had to complete six laps of a supersprint triathlon course. Each lap consisted of a 200-metre swim in the lake, a 5.3-kilometre bike ride of two laps round the water's edge, and a 1.5-kilometre run. In other words, six swims, six bike sections and six runs, a staggering 18 sections. Imagine the scene with up to half a dozen people in each team: it was utterly chaotic. Kit was everywhere – hundreds of bikes, wetsuits and helmets all cluttering the gigantic transition area.

The most amusing thing about the rules – or lack of rules – was that as long as the swims, bikes and runs were completed in that sequence over and over until all 18 sections were finished, the team members could do any section they wanted. All they had to do was make sure the timing chip was handed over to the next competitor at every swap. It meant the super-competitive teams could all play to their strengths and choose their top swimmer to do all the swims, for example. At the other end of the scale, if someone didn't fancy doing the running, they didn't have to; someone else could do it in their place.

Our team was an eclectic bunch.

The team leader was *Comic Relief*'s Kevin Cahill, who had learned to swim only a year earlier, in order to take part in a triathlon. He had now persuaded two members of the *Comic Relief* office staff, neither of whom had ever done a triathlon before, to join us. We were also joined by Professor Greg Whyte, a World Championship silver medallist in the Modern Pentathlon, and his wife, Penny. They were both super-fast. Whyte is one of the world's leading sports psychologists, and successfully coached Davina McCall, Eddie Izzard and David Walliams through their epic challenges for *Comic Relief*.

Kevin decided we would all do a swim, bike and a run – but not necessarily in sequence, which would allow us a rest in between. Having seen Greg dart like a dolphin through the water, I would have made him do every single swim, but that day was not about the winning, just about the excitement of taking part.

Because the rules allowed it, and to make matters more challenging for me, I competed in two teams that day. My younger brother, Mark, was also running a team, and he wanted me in it. We worked out that if I timed it right I could run between the two teams – and I should be able to complete quite a few of their sections too.

The camaraderie was amazing, and so were the combinations. Every team seemed to be approaching the competition differently. Once the race started, it was like a study in motion: a busy triathlon circus with people running in and out of transition, pulling off timing chips, passing them one to another, forgetting things, turning back, starting all over again, and cheering encouragement.

The highlight of the day was when the last runner in every team finally finished: the whole team waited on the side of the running course and then everyone ran the last 100 metres together, for a celebratory photo crossing the line, hands linked and held high in the air. I loved the whole day, loved being a part of it and seeing hundreds of people relishing the sport I love and having great fun doing it.

Some of my most enjoyable races have been competing as part of a family relay. With my brother, Mark, and my husband, David, I have taken part twice in the JLL Property Triathlon North, which is held every year right outside my *BBC Breakfast* office in

Salford. Competing there brings juggling work and triathlon to a whole new level.

Transition is set up in the piazza in MediaCity, just below our studios, so when I arrive at the office at 4.50 a.m. I walk past the empty bike racks, all set up and ready to go. By the time I finish on air at 9.15 a.m. the race is pretty much in full swing, and it is fantastic to watch from outside the studio as triathletes, fresh out of the water in Salford Quays, run towards my office in their wetsuits, change quickly and then zoom out on their bikes right in front of the BBC entrance.

The first time we competed was in 2015, the year I qualified for the Great Britain team, so we agreed that I needed race practice on my bike and that anyway I would probably be the fastest of the three of us on two wheels. Mark, who is super-fast, volunteered to take on the 750-metre swim, and David took on my least favourite discipline, the run.

The run-up to the race had been great, and made my training much more fun. For once, rather than always running on my own, David had been accompanying Waffle and me as part of his preparation. During the early summer months, we enjoyed a fantastic routine: a couple of days a week, when I got home from work, we both put our trainers on to go for a jog by the river with a delighted Labrador. I knew that David would do us proud on the day: he is extremely determined, and though unable to run the distances that I can, is much faster on a shorter course.

For us, entering the race was supposed to be about having a laugh, but when the morning of the race arrived we were all ridiculously nervous, not wanting to be the one that let the team down. As always, I was pushing the edges of logistical possibilities, and finished presenting *Breakfast* only about 15 minutes before Mark was due to start in the water. I made a very quick change out of my smart presenting clothes in the ladies' loo, tied my hair in a ponytail and dashed down to the start. There I found the two of them waiting by my bike, fidgeting apprehensively and ready to go.

As David and I walked Mark down to the start he was trying to talk down his swimming abilities, but we were both optimistic for him. True to form, he got us off to a cracking start, cutting through the water seemingly without effort. I had to dash back to my bike to be ready when he came out. He did brilliantly, running into transition second in our wave.

It was surreal but exhilarating to leap on to my bike in the shadows of the studio, and head out of the piazza at breakneck speed. The 20-kilometre bike ride was five exhilarating laps, on a cordoned-off section of road with a wonderfully smooth surface. The only problem was, we all had to count our own laps. That might sound simple, but when you are concentrating on staying safe on the road and pedalling as fast as you can, you can easily get confused. Thankfully, David and Mark had that covered, taking it in turns to stand at the top of the course and shout at me every time I finished a lap.

I managed to overtake a few riders on the way, and arrived in transition out of breath but with a huge grin on my face, to hand the timing chip as quickly as I could to David. He set off like a steam train on the 5-kilometre run – and was so fast that Mark and I, who were chatting while waiting to cheer him on, entirely missed him as he finished his first lap of three. I knew he would be furious that we weren't concentrating, so on the second lap we cheered extra loudly.

David would be quick, I knew, but he surpassed all our expectations. He absolutely stormed it with a cracking time of 21 minutes, 45 seconds. Despite all my training, I can still only dream of such a time. As we all crossed the finish line together, I was quite concerned, though: he could hardly breathe, let alone talk. To my relief, he recovered quickly and we all collapsed in a heap by the *Blue Peter* Garden, joining dozens of other triathletes sharing the post-race euphoria, drinking beer and chatting through the best bits of the day. We had come sixth out of 64 mixed relay teams – not bad at all.

The following year, we decided to race as a team again. This time, though, David was injured and couldn't do the run, so we mixed up the disciplines and, without meaning to, made it much more competitive for ourselves. I took the swim, David the bike and Mark the run. Once again, we all loved the day, but this time we had the added pressure of being able to compare our times against each other.

Given that I do a lot more cycling than David, I was hoping my bike ride would be faster than his. Thank goodness it was! I had finished mine in 35.50 and he now managed 37.23, claiming he was only slower because he had a stitch.

Mark was adamant that I wouldn't beat his swim. I didn't think I would either, but neither of us had factored in all the training and technique practice I had done. So, when I came out of the water with a time of 12 minutes, 36 seconds for the 750 metres, soundly beating him by 1 minute, 20 seconds, he was infuriated. That was compounded by his 5-kilometre run time of 23.13, which was nearly two minutes slower than David's result the year before.

Nearly a year on from the race, Mark is still muttering about changes to the course, and the fact that his swim and run were definitely longer than ours. We just tell him to look at the results! There is nothing quite like a bit of silly sibling rivalry.

We were hoping to race again this year, and change all the disciplines around again, but Mark was – very conveniently – away on holiday. I have told him there is always next year, and by then I should have had more time to speed up my run.

In my experience, triathlon relays are a brilliant way to spice up the sport, and it is not just amateurs like me who enjoy them. At the 2014 Commonwealth Games in Glasgow, the formidable English quartet of Vicky Holland, Jonathan Brownlee, Jodie Stimpson and Alistair Brownlee won gold in the mixed relay, and at the 2020 Summer Olympics in Tokyo, mixed relay will be one of the events.

For the elite mixed relay, there are teams of four: two men and two women. Each member of the team completes a supersprint triathlon before tagging the next member of the team, and so on, until they have all finished. Supersprint is normally a 300-metre swim, 7.5 kilometre cycle and a 1.5 kilometre run. I watched it up close after finishing the European Championships in Lisbon, and it is incredibly fast, dynamic, and exciting to watch as a spectator.

I can't wait to see it at the Olympics.

CHAPTER 26

BEING COMPETITIVE

'I would love to win, if it ever happened, but winning, and beating other people, is not my motivation.'

One of the questions I have thought about a great deal during my triathlon adventure is whether I am 'competitive', and what that description really means in the 21st century.

I am sure that if I didn't have a competitive streak, I wouldn't be sitting on the *BBC Breakfast* sofa or competing in triathlon World Championships. Being described as competitive worries me, though. It sounds negative, a pejorative term with ugly undertones. I suppose this might reflect my own preconceptions about what 'competitive' means, and what I think is implied by saying I'm a 'competitive' woman.

It makes me wonder why it seems OK – even more than that, a good thing – to describe a man as competitive, whether at work or in sport. Why does 'competitive' have positive connotations for a man and negative implications for a woman? And if being competitive means that you strive to be good at what you do, is that a bad thing?

When someone says, 'Louise, you are so competitive', I assume they think I want to win at all costs, to the detriment of other people, with no concern or empathy for anyone else. That's not the case. I would love to win, if it ever happened, but winning, and beating other people, is not my motivation. So, does that mean I am still competitive? I think if I were truly competitive, I would have packed up my tri suit by now and given it all up. The reality is, I am never going to be the winner. That's not why I do it, which is why I haven't.

There are times, of course, when I am fiercely competitive. That seminal moment in the Velodrome, for example, when Bill Turnbull said he couldn't be beaten by a girl, was like a red rag to a bull. After he said that, there was no way I wasn't going to try my absolute hardest to beat him. I will also admit that if I ever find myself in a sprint finish in a swim or a run, and have anything left in my energy tank, I always dig deep, push hard and try to be first to cross the line. But those victories are not the reason I start the race. Winning is not my main motivation.

There are two things that motivate me. Firstly, doing something I love; and secondly, striving to do it better. That doesn't mean having to, or even wanting to, triumph over anyone else. It is a competition or battle with myself.

My job at *BBC Breakfast* and taking part in triathlon are both examples of this.

I love my job. From the age of five, I have loved recounting stories and asking questions. So much so that when I started to tell my family one of my endless tales, my parents would roll their eyes, groan and ask my sister, Nikki, to let them know when it was all over. Four decades later, I am still doing what I loved to do then, telling people about the latest news stories and asking questions, trying to find out why things happen.

So, I don't present *BBC Breakfast* because I am competitive, I present it because I love it. I am part of a team that is constantly striving to make the programme as good as it can possibly be. That is what is important to me: to be always trying to improve myself and at the same time help make the programme better.

With triathlon, it is a similar story.

I race because I love racing. I love the camaraderie, standing at the start surrounded by other competitors, nervous and excited, in anticipation of the adventure. I love going as fast as I physically can, gliding through the water, speeding along on my bike, and even battling through the pain barrier on the run. I love the wave of adrenaline and endorphins after pushing myself hard and trying my absolute best.

I never start the race because I want to win. I start it because I love taking part. The only person I am really competing against is myself. I am always striving to get a little better, race a little faster, bring down my times. If I beat someone else along the way, that is fun, but only incidental.

So, to come back to that question: 'Am I competitive?', the honest answer is: Yes. What I would like to do, though, is remove some of the toxin surrounding the use of the word. Try as I might, I can never find the perfect English word to describe what motivates me, but there is a perfect one in Spanish: *voluntad*. Literally, it means willpower. The way the Spanish tend to use it, I think it translates better as 'wanting to do it'. In my mind, *voluntad* means you can do anything you set your mind to, without having to push other people out of the way. *Voluntad*, as I see it, is a positive and powerful mix of determination, focus and drive.

If someone said, 'Louise, you have so much *voluntad*', I would feel immensely proud and flattered. Trouble is, I don't suppose I'll ever be able to slip the word into an English dictionary.

CHAPTER 27

BUTTERFLIES AND STAGE FRIGHT

'I turn from being a supremely able, happy-go-lucky multitasker into a shambolic and chaotic scatterbrain.'

I'm scared, I can't breathe, I can't do this, I don't want to do this, I am walking away right now!

I was about to read a one-minute news bulletin, at 11 o'clock in the morning, for my very first time on BBC One, and I was in a blind panic.

'Cue Louise,' shouted my friend and director, Chris Cook, down my earpiece.

Miraculously, the words 'Good morning, I'm Louise Minchin and these are the headlines' tumbled breathlessly out of my dry mouth. I'd done it!

For me, stage fright feels like being overpowered in a tsunami of negative thoughts that freeze me with fear. I have had full-blown stage fright only a couple of times. Each time, although I had been nervous, with butterflies churning round my stomach,

I had no inkling that I was about to be paralysed with panic. It seems to come from nowhere.

I have always suffered from nerves, right from the day I took part in my first swimming race. Even now, decades later, when I am getting ready for a race, they still affect me, and I still don't like the way they make me feel: jittery, hot, sweaty, nauseous, heart racing, and like my intestines are tied in knots being twisted by a giant. When I am in the grip of a nervous panic, it doesn't just affect me physically, my behaviour changes too.

David says that when I am nervous pre-race, I turn from being a supremely able, happy-go-lucky multitasker into a shambolic and chaotic scatterbrain. He says it's not a pretty picture. I can't concentrate, can't focus, can't respond to questions, and start talking utter gibberish. Luckily for me, he is brilliant at coping with it. He is not offended by my abruptness, and just takes over the logistics, going through every detail and all the checklists I have written with military precision. Left to my own devices, I am very likely to forget something crucial, and frequently have.

Dealing with pre-race nerves is a struggle, and I don't think that the heebie-jeebies will ever leave me. What I try to do now is embrace them and accept that, as long as I can keep them under control and the anxiety doesn't turn into full-blown stage fright, they are a good thing for both my job and in triathlon.

A couple of years ago, I had a breakthrough.

I was presenting *BBC Breakfast* with Dan Walker, and we were trying to do something that at first seemed to be impossible, even slightly ridiculous. We were attempting to power a remote-controlled car using only our thoughts. Yes, really! If this technology can be developed, the hope is that people with spinal injuries will in the future be able to control their wheelchairs using their brainwaves.

That's why I found myself, live on national television, wearing a headset scanning my brain. The extraordinary-looking contraptions were connected to a giant Scalextric track with two cars on it. In theory, the energy supplied from our brainwaves would power the cars. To me, this seemed inconceivable – and, just as I presumed, my car wouldn't move a millimetre. Not at first, anyway. Then the technician in charge explained that what I needed to do was *not* to think, but just calm my thoughts down to a standstill. According to the theory, my brainwaves would then move faster, and so would the electric car.

For some reason, my mind went back to that Zen-like moment I had experienced swimming with jellyfish in the docks in Liverpool, seeing them suspended in the deep blue water and amazed by their beauty. Visualising them, I remembered how peaceful I felt at the time. My heart stopped racing and my breathing slowed down, along with my thoughts. Immediately, the car shot off, screeching round the corners at astonishing speeds – so fast, in fact, that it hurtled off the tracks. I couldn't believe it.

That was a revelation to me. Till then, I had no concept just how powerful a tool visualisation could be. Now I return to that image often, to deal with anxiety. Whenever I feel nerves beginning to overwhelm me, I close my eyes for a second, take a couple of breaths and think about how serene I felt watching those jellyfish. When I open my eyes again, I am calm, focused and ready for anything.

This worked brilliantly in the seconds before I was due to go on stage at Wembley Arena, in front of 8,000 people. Along with Jeremy Vine, I was about to present a minute-by-minute documentary to commemorate the anniversary of England winning the 1966 World Cup.

I was under a huge amount of pressure. The programme was going out live on BBC Radio 2 and being simulcast in cinemas around the UK. We were working with an orchestra, half a dozen bands, and a handful of actors, including Martin Freeman, star of *Sherlock* and *The Hobbit*. The actors were playing different parts, from the Queen to Bobby Moore and Geoff Hurst. I had an incredibly complicated and intricate script, which required me to be very precise, and to get my words, timings and cues exactly right. This was a hugely ambitious programme, and if I got so much as one word or cue wrong, the whole programme could come stumbling to a dramatic halt – and it would be all my fault.

In the hours leading up to the simulcast, I was doing OK; chatting happily with singer-songwriter Sophie Ellis-Bextor in our shared dressing room, and calmly going through my lines. Until, that is, the floor manager beckoned to Jeremy and me to make our entrance on to the stage. I felt myself turn ice-cold with anxiety, and my heart leap – sensations made a hundred times worse by seeing that even the seasoned actor Martin Freeman, standing next to me, looked a touch nervous.

A wave of panic rolled over me, but for the first time, instead of succumbing to it, I closed my eyes and visualised those jellyfish, just for a moment. The moment I opened my eyes I was absolutely fine and completely focused. I knew that whatever happened, I was going to be OK, I could nail it. What's more, it was going to be great fun too.

Before that breakthrough, and even now, I try lots of different ways to cope with nerves, both at work and before races.

The most effective thing for me is to be as organised as I possibly can be, leaving as little as possible to chance. There is less room for silly errors if I have been meticulous in my preparation.

For triathlons, there will usually be a race briefing the day before the competition. I will always try to go because I find them incredibly helpful. I often pick up golden nuggets of information that are relevant for that particular course. Not only is it helpful on the day, but it helps to calm me down in the hours leading up to it, as I now have a better idea of what lies ahead.

The night before the European Championships in Lisbon, the officials said that the exit from the swim was up a steep ramp and likely to be slippery. Somehow I remembered and, sure enough, when I scrabbled on to my feet on the sharp incline, I slowed down when others didn't, and watched, horrified, as several fellow competitors fell awkwardly on to the hard concrete.

Nor do I just rely on official information: a little local knowledge can go a very long way.

In those nervy moments when I am standing in my wetsuit surrounded by other triathletes about to get into the water, I will often chat to people, particularly if I discover that they live there or have raced the course before. Just before I ran into the choppy sea in a race in Lanzarote, I asked a seasoned competitor the best way to swim the course, and he pointed out which buildings I should head towards. Thank goodness he did! When I dived into the sea, the water was so rough I couldn't catch sight of the huge fluorescent buoys we were meant to be turning around. I followed his instructions, using the buildings as sighting points, and when everyone set off in a different direction, headed my own way. I had a cracking swim and, for the first and probably the last time in my life, beat my own coach, Claire, by five seconds out of the water.

One of my biggest struggles with nerves used to be trying to sleep the night before a race. Writing a proper kit list has helped enormously, but it is not a cure-all. I still get nervous, but if I can't doze off, I very slowly go through the race plan, visualising every moment right from the start and answering a list of questions.

How am I going to lay out my kit in transition? Is the swim a beach start or deep-water start? How long is the run to the bike from the swim exit? Is it carpet or gravel? What order am I going to take off my wetsuit, put on my helmet and sunglasses? Where is the mount line for my bike? I go through the list in such intricate detail that by the time I imagine myself actually getting on the bike, I have bored myself to sleep. For me it is like a triathlete's version of counting sheep.

After years of battling with nerves, I have realised that apprehension is a good thing as long as I can control it.

The nerves mean that I prepare properly, get organised, think things through. They mean that I am 100 per cent ready, focused both physically and mentally for the moment the transmission light goes red, or the whistle blows. Nerves are a necessary part of trying hard.

After I have read the first headline or swum the first 100 metres, the nerves disappear into the ether as if they had never existed – I am lost in the moment, enjoying what I set out to do.

Maybe the nerves were just excitement, after all.

CHAPTER 28

TEAM MINCHIN

'Winning isn't everything, and losing should never stop you trying.'

'Mummy, I really respect what you do.'

I was taken aback by the comment from my eldest daughter, Mia.

It was a beautiful day, and we were ambling in the sunshine across Queens Wharf in Liverpool, the bridge that crosses the point where the Queens Dock and Wapping Dock meet each other. Many years before, in the 1800s, it would have been the scene of a bustling Victorian shipping hub trading in brandy, cotton, tea, silk, tobacco and sugar. Now, the towering granite and iron warehouses are filled with restaurants, hotels and apartments.

We were on our way to do some retail therapy in Liverpool ONE, and chatting about triathlon. I had been reminiscing about the last time I had been near that bridge, racing in the then blueish but now cold grey waters below us, and then falling off my bike as I came into transition. I had hauled myself up and, despite a bloodied knee and elbow, went on to win my age group for the first time.

I don't really know what I had expected her to say, and was surprised to hear that she admired me – for my bravery, my enthusiasm and my determination.

I have had more than a few emotional moments during my triathlon career, but Mia's words are right at the top.

Way back when my triathlon adventure first began, I read some research about girls and their participation in sport, published by Sport England. Their findings showed that when a mother participated in weekly sport, their daughters were much more likely to participate in sport too. I was struck by the fact that it was the mums being active, and not the dads, that seemed to make the difference.

The research had a profound impact on me. I really wanted my daughters to avoid the mistake I had made, and deeply regret, giving up sport in my teenage years. The research showed me that my example could have a direct impact on their decisions. If I wanted to encourage them to continue with sport as part of their life, it had to be part of mine. I had to lead by example. I had to get up and get out there to show them that sport isn't something that only dads or boys do. It's something we can all do. I would have to adopt the *This Girl Can* approach to sport.

When Mia made clear her respect for me, suddenly all those months of going on runs when I didn't want to, immersing myself in cold water in a lake when I would rather have been in a hot bath, sweating away on my turbo when I could have been sitting on the sofa watching TV – all of those months made sense. Every second, minute and hour spent trying had value. A value measured in the respect of my teenager. That moment on the bridge brought tears to my eyes.

Since then, I have asked her for more thoughts about my triathlon adventures. Not only does she respect me, but it turns out she is inspired by me too – and once again, it's not for the reasons I had imagined. It's not because I have qualified for and competed in the World and European Championships.

It's because, she explains, I have stuck at something even though I am not very good.

When she first said that, I have to be honest: I was taken aback. *Not very good? What does she mean? I have represented my country. How is that 'not very good'?*

On reflection, though – and once I'd put my umbrage aside – I realised she makes a very good point, one that reinforces my conviction that all the effort and hundreds of hours of training have been worthwhile.

She has been witness to my endless struggles. She has seen that when I finish last in a 10-mile time trial on my bike, I don't let it demoralise or stop me, I will always go back to have another go. When I am the slowest in a run session on the athletics track, I am not embarrassed, I don't give up, I go back and try again.

Where I come or how I do is irrelevant to her. It is the fact that I try, and keep on trying, sticking with it in the face of disappointments and mistakes, that is important to her.

I realise that my tenacity has shown her that there is a value in effort, that winning isn't everything, and losing should never stop you trying. I have dared to try – and I hope that my efforts will encourage her too.

When I ask whether my efforts will inspire her to continue with sport into adulthood, she gives a definite yes. She is unlikely to try triathlon, but sport – whether it is running with the dog, bashing a tennis ball or going to the gym – is important to her, for her sense of well-being. She knows she doesn't need to win or be the best to enjoy it.

My younger daughter, Scarlett, was only eight when I started triathlon, and she can hardly remember life before there was a racing bike cluttering up the hall or I was shouting up the stairs: 'Does anyone want to come for a run?', or she was encouraging me from the shoreline as I braced myself for yet another swim in the river.

I can picture her quite clearly on my first ever race, jogging along beside me on that painful 5-kilometre run on the Meadows in Chester. She was wrapped up in a bright red puffy coat, blonde hair tied in a ponytail, shouting: 'Come on, Mummy, you are amazing, you can do this.'

It was a memorable and touching moment. Total role reversal: she, my young daughter, was encouraging me, her mother. She was right, too. I could do it – but only because my optimistic eight-year-old was there to support me.

She has always been supremely reassuring and enthusiastic during my races, and despite any disasters. I love hearing her encouraging comments as I make a mess of transition, her wide smiles and huge hugs when I finish, and the way she always says 'Well done, Mummy', no matter where I have come and however long I took. Like Mia, she doesn't care about the medals either, and says she is proud and happy for me because she can see me doing something I really love.

For teenage daughters, there are also unexpected benefits in having a mum who is a triathlete.

When I am on the verge of nagging, Scarlett in particular is quick to spot it and will nag me too. She knows about my terrible tendency to put off a bike ride, a run or a swim – and also knows that once I have been out to exercise, I am much more relaxed, less stressed and far less likely to be on their case about homework or tidying their rooms.

They frequently say to me, 'Mummy, go on, go out for a run, you know you will love it. Why don't you go for a swim? You know you will feel better.'

I often do exactly as they suggest, and the best thing is that they are right, I do feel a million times better. The bonus from their point of view is that they have time left to their own devices (literally). As for me, I often find that when I get back, their homework is finished and their rooms are tidier too.

There is no doubt that I couldn't compete without the support of my whole family.

I owe much to my husband. David is the backbone and driving force of Team Minchin, as well as the official chief cheerleader and logistics manager. Without his support, I couldn't do it. I would probably still be languishing in an occasional trip to the pool and a half-hearted run with the dog. He knows how important it is to me, for two key reasons – as an effective means of mentally disengaging from work and because I get a massive kick out of competing. To help me do both, he is tirelessly and fiercely supportive.

He helps me in a hundred different ways, whether it is cycling alongside me into the Welsh hills, driving me in the early hours to a competition, double-checking that I have checked my checklist, helping me fix a problem with my bike, finding some crucial piece of equipment I have misplaced in a pre-race panic, and calming me down when I am jittery with nervous apprehension. Whatever I need, whatever the problem is, he is always there to calm me down and sort me out.

The importance of his support is never more obvious than on race-day. By looking after the girls, and taking charge of all the other logistics, he leaves me completely free to focus on getting ready for the race.

Thanks to David, race-day is a stress-free zone. I am extremely lucky. Without him, the wheels would have come off my triathlon experience a long time ago.

While he is impressed by my levels of determination and proud of what I have achieved, he is also my biggest critic. It might be painful to hear what he has to say, but I have to concede that he often has a point.

For example, when we are out for a run, he will jog along beside me and tell me I could sharpen up my running technique. Anyone who has seen me run can probably agree, and although I have put a huge amount of effort into trying to fix it, there is still a long way to go.

I don't like it when he says it, but I know he is right.

When we are doing some post-race analysis, he sometimes says that he thinks I have left something in the tank, that I could have tried a little harder. Though I don't like to admit it, he has a point there, too. I am often holding back – scared that if I don't, I might not finish.

Even in the swim, I worry that I shouldn't try too hard, shouldn't get too out of breath, that if I do try and swim even faster I won't make it to the end.

He says he pushes me because I need pushing, and that I don't realise what I am capable of achieving. His honesty is a wonderful asset and a major reason I have improved as a triathlete.

That leaves me with some philosophical questions.

Do I want to go faster? Is what I have achieved enough already? Am I too scared to try any harder? Does pushing myself stop me from enjoying myself? What really matters?

As yet, I am not sure that I have the answers. What I do know is that family is everything. Without their love and support, none of it would have been possible.

CHAPTER 29

THE PERFECT TRAINING PARTNER

'Every run we have done together has felt shorter, easier, and more like fun.'

Without the unfailing support of my best, most loyal and dedicated training partner, I would never have made it into the Great Britain team. She is effusive in her enthusiasm, unfailing in her encouragement, never lets me down by having better plans, and is ready at any hour of the day, seven days a week, to accompany me on a run.

She is, of course, my golden Labrador, Waffle.

When this blonde, cuddly and somewhat clumsy puppy arrived, with her hazel brown eyes and a waggy tail, we all fell in love with her instantly. Five years later she is an integral, much loved part of our family – and, as it has turned out, a wonderful and inspiring training companion.

Ever since she was four years old, my eldest daughter, Mia, wanted to have a dog. At the time, we lived in Wandsworth in south London, and I thought a busy city wasn't a good place for a dog to live. It didn't seem fair on an animal to have little access to outside space and only the pavements to pound.

But Mia wasn't prepared to take no for an answer, and started an endless onslaught of requests. 'Please, Mummy, can we have a dog?' 'Why can't we have a dog, Mummy?' 'I promise I will look after it, Mummy. Please!' 'I would love to have a dog, Mummy, please!'

She wouldn't let it go. One day, worn down by her incessant mantra, instead of saying no, I promised that when she was 11, I would make her wish come true, she could have a dog. At the time, I picked 11 only because it was a random number and so far ahead that I assumed she would forget all about it. I underestimated her. She didn't forget, not for one day, and I lost count of the times she reminded me of my promise. 'Remember, you promised I could have a dog when I was 11.'

As luck would have it, Mia's 11th birthday coincided with the summer we moved to the north-west with *BBC Breakfast.* Like many 11-year-olds faced with a life-changing move, Mia wasn't particularly enamoured by the idea that we should leave the house she had always known, change schools, and live somewhere we had never even visited before and where we didn't know anyone.

As part of selling her the benefits of such a move, I finally had to relent and promise her that we would get a dog. It was an unashamed piece of parental bribery.

That's why Waffle duly arrived, in September 2012, and I am so happy she did.

She was nine weeks old when she reached our house, after a long car journey from Somerset, wrapped up in a blanket on Scarlett's knee. Waffle was still wobbly on her oversized paws, and her soft skin looked like an ill-fitting coat, three sizes too big for her.

Right from the start she was inquisitive, cuddly and affectionate, and we couldn't help but adore her and return her affection, smothering her with love.

Waffle's arrival also coincided with my first tentative steps into triathlon, and by the time she was about a year old, we were running together on a regular basis. I was careful to start slowly and take her for only short distances at first. Labradors can have problems with their hips and it's not advisable to run too far with them before they are about two years old. But over the weeks and months, and now years, we have got stronger and fitter together.

Since those early days of slow, short runs, when she was still nervous and easily spooked by another dog or even by a duck splashing down on the river, I can't count how many miles we have covered together.

When I run with her, it is as if we are attached by an invisible lead, which only we know is there.

One thing never changes, though. She will always be carrying something in her mouth. It might be a stick she found under a tree, or a tennis ball lost by another dog and sniffed out from its hiding place deep in the undergrowth with her sensitive nose. She always needs to be carrying something.

Our favourite place to run is near home, along the banks of the River Dee. When we are running alongside the water's edge, she always positions herself about five metres ahead of me, at an easy pace, ears pricked, tail up, on the alert for any danger, like a trail-blazing pacemaker. She takes the duties she has assumed as my personal bodyguard very seriously. If she sees another dog, walker or runner ahead, she will drop back to trot by my side and warn me. Going past them, she won't take a blind bit of notice, won't stop and sniff, or let someone pat her; she seems to think her job is to stick right beside me, watching out for me.

She is so in tune with me, that if I slow my pace she slows down too. Without even glancing back to see what I am up to, she readjusts her pace to match mine, and to make sure the invisible lead between us stays the same length. If I want her to change direction, all I have to do is say her name, and point at where I want to go, and she heads off wherever I have pointed.

Having her as my training partner has been very motivational. There is not a day that goes by when she wouldn't like to go for a run, and the weather is no barrier. Whether it is freezing, pouring or just plain miserable, she will always be grateful when she sees me putting my trainers on.

I love her myriad ways of encouraging me to go out.

If I am writing or trying to wade through emails, she will sit near my feet, head between her paws, looking up with her sandy brown eyes and gently wagging her tail, with her top lip curling as if she was trying to smile and say, *Please, come on, you know I want to go out.* Or she might wander over and quietly nudge my leg with her wet nose, to remind me, *I am here, I am ready, come on! You know we can do this.*

She knows that her best chance for a run is when I get back home from *BBC Breakfast*, and if she can be persuasive enough I will probably take her out. As soon as she hears me open the door on my return, she barks loudly, rushes about in search of my running shoes, and when she has found one she brings it to me in hope and expectation while wildly leaping around.

When I relent and put on my running kit, her enthusiasm can reach desperate levels. She is beside herself with exuberance, whining hysterically, dashing round in tight circles, and jumping up on her hind legs, as if the cool kitchen tiles were hot coals burning her paws.

Without Waffle, there is no question that I would have found all the running I have had to do much harder. We have spent so many happy hours together, and her companionship has meant that every run we have done together has felt shorter, easier and more like fun. Without her, those countless hours of training would have felt almost impossible, and I am immensely grateful for her dedication to the cause.

Without her, I doubt I would have made the team.

CHAPTER 30

PUSHING YOURSELF

'If you're not nervous, it means it doesn't matter to you, it's not important and you're not going to fire up the adrenaline.'

Paula Radcliffe, six-time world champion and marathon world record holder

When I look back over the last few years and all the adventures in triathlon, I realise that there have been a couple of moments when I have found myself face to face with overwhelming fear and self-doubt, and paralysed by negativity. In those moments, the whole endeavour has seemed dangerous, deeply stupid, and utterly pointless.

I vividly remember the feeling of being locked in a hot, claustrophobic Portaloo in Fountains Abbey, breathing fast, sweating profusely and refusing to race. It felt terrifying at the time. Likewise, I can remember the deafening, debilitating thoughts at the start of the 10-kilometre run at the Dambuster Triathlon, where I surpassed my expectations and went on to qualify for the World Championships.

What is the psychology behind those moments? Am I alone in feeling like that? Are the experiences in any way instructive and even helpful in the long term? Do elite athletes suffer the same way? Or do they have some magic gene that keeps them cool, calm and collected under pressure?

To get to the bottom of those questions, I talked to the lead psychologist at British Cycling, Dr Ruth Anderson. She has worked in sport psychology for years, helping athletes all over the world achieve their potential and win gold medals. In 2016 she went to the Summer Olympics in Rio with the British Cycling Team, working with the likes of the track cyclists Jason Kenny and Laura Trott.

First, we talked about the paralysing fright I experienced behind the closed doors of that Portaloo. That, she said, was a classic example of the fight-or-flight response. I was experiencing both a physical and psychological reaction to what at the time appeared to be a very real threat:

'Physiologically, when you are nervous your heart is racing, your muscles start to get tense, some people will shake. Your blood pressure will increase, although you won't be able to feel it. Some people might feel butterflies in their tummy or physically sick. And you may notice a shortness of breath. Cognitively what is happening, your mind could be racing, you may be overthinking, likely to have difficulty making decisions with excess worry, self-doubt and the *what if?* questions.'

I was doing the triathlon for fun, but right then and there in the Portaloo it didn't feel fun at all. I felt out of control. Again, according to Ruth, this is a normal and natural response:

'You had voluntarily put yourself under extreme pressure, challenging yourself, taking a risk and making yourself vulnerable to failure, and that had made you extremely anxious.'

Ruth reassured me I am not alone in that reaction. Lots of people who choose to put themselves in extremely challenging situations, even successful Olympic athletes, come to those crunch moments and experience a fight-or-flight response.

It's human – and what is crucial is how you respond.

In that moment, hiding in the Portaloo, I had two stark choices. *Either* I could back away from the situation, withdraw from the triathlon and go home a little bit ashamed, with a furious family *or* I could choose to fight the anxiety, stand my ground, push through it and race. I was in full flight mode, and mustered the alternative fight response only with the help of my daughter Mia, who was knocking frantically on the door and saying the right thing at the right time: 'Get in the water!' That simple instruction forced me to pull myself together, focus and get my head back in the game.

Ruth Anderson says that everyone is the same:

'Most successful athletes have been through key moments like that, because as the pressure increases your anxiety increases and people will react differently at different times. Some athletes might have difficulties early on in managing anxiety; others, it will be later on – but everyone has it. Some people think that a confident athlete will not get anxious, but everyone has anxiety because that is what pressure does: it generates anxiety. And so you need to learn how you respond when anxious and learn strategies which help you constantly push through it, so you can achieve at your best.'

Even marathon runner Paula Radcliffe, a world record holder, has been through a moment of incapacitating anxiety early on in her running career:

'I remember when I was 13 or 14 and I did my first big event. I remember being so nervous I was almost physically sick beforehand and my dad took me aside, saying, look, this is meant to be fun, it's meant to be something you do because you enjoy it. If you get that sick, I'm not going to bring you to races anymore, so you need to get this under control.'

Paula says that for her, and myself, it was our response in that moment that really mattered, the choice we made, not where we came in the race. Paula didn't win, nor did she expect to. She came 14th, and afterwards she never felt that nervous again.

Ruth again: 'It doesn't feel like it at the time, because the emotion and the feeling is so overwhelming, but it is a choice. You have to make that decision to push through. Talk to your coach, talk to your family, it doesn't matter how you do it, just that you are able to do it.'

If you can get through it, the results of facing your anxiety head-on are very significant, according to Ruth – and much more important to future successes than winning a particular race.

'If you choose to face the anxiety, fight it, you will know in the future that however nervous you get, you do have the capacity to push through.'

Had I backed down that day at Fountains Abbey, hung my head in shame, peeled off my wetsuit, picked up my bike and gone home, I would most likely never have raced again. Instead, what I learned was that, even if I feel sick with nerves, overwhelmed by them, paralysed by them, it doesn't matter. I can deal with it, and race anyway.

That was a seminal moment, a turning point – and, like Paula, I have never felt so nervous again.

'Once you have pushed through it, you start to develop a better tolerance for how you cope with those challenging situations. And that is the only way you can keep challenging yourself and achieve at a high level, if you are willing to do that.'

That's the bad side of performance anxiety. On the upside, it shouldn't be forgotten that nerves, as long as they are kept under control, can enhance your performance.

As Paula explains: 'If you're not nervous, it means it doesn't matter to you, it's not important and you're not going to fire up the adrenaline.'

The other key moment in my triathlon journey was that collision with self-doubt that nearly stopped me from qualifying for the World Championships in Chicago. I often hear the voices of self-doubt, but that day they were a cacophony.

Paula is very open about suffering similar experiences:

'I definitely found the hardest time to manage nerves-wise was the night before when you go to sleep, because you're not actually doing anything to burn off the adrenaline, you're not warming up. Once you start warming up, you can start getting it all under control. So I had to find techniques to kind of escape from that feeling of *Oh my God, this is a really important race for me. What if I don't run it right? What if I'm not feeling good tomorrow?* My way of distracting myself was to carry books around and just bury myself in a book somewhere.'

Non Stanford, a World Champion triathlete, says it is in the hour before a race, when she is getting ready and organising her kit in transition, that she is at her most nervous and starts to seriously question her lifestyle choices.

Even Sir Bradley Wiggins, five-time Olympic gold-medal-winning cyclist and the first Briton to win the Tour de France, says he has moments of anxiety and self-doubt. He told me that for him, these are most intense during the couple of hours before a race, particularly in the febrile atmosphere of a velodrome. The huge pressure of knowing all the hard work and effort of four years comes down to just that moment makes him start to worry with thoughts like, *What if it all goes wrong and I mess it up at the start line?*

Again, according to Ruth, British Cycling's lead psychologist, it is all perfectly normal performance anxiety.

'There is not a gold medallist that I have worked with that hasn't had doubts in their ability at different times. Everyone has the voice in their head. There is a myth that some elite athletes won't have that voice of doubt in their head, or they won't at some point have some doubt in their ability. Everyone does, we are all human. What elite athletes learn to do is develop the skill to be able to control their thinking under pressure.'

That is echoed by many of the successful athletes I have spoken to, but what seems different from their experiences and mine as an amateur athlete is that once the starting gun goes for them, all the doubts disappear into the ether as if they never existed, and they are able to get on with the race free from anxiety.

So, why do my doubts resurface, in the middle or towards the end of a triathlon? Is there anything I can do about it?

Ruth believes this is down to concentration levels and focus. Unless you are like Paula Radcliffe and your years of competing have trained you not to let your thoughts wander, it is likely to happen when you are struggling physically and have become distracted by pain or fatigue.

'Those invasive thoughts and self-doubt are totally normal and natural, especially in a long and multi-discipline event like triathlon, where you have to think differently for every event. You can only hold your concentration and attention for a certain amount of time. You can't focus for such a long length of time; it is just not realistic. The danger is, if you let the thoughts sit in your mind, they will start influencing what you do, you will start finding evidence for them, and then it will affect your race.'

In the excruciatingly hard 10 kilometres running along Rutland Water, that was exactly what was happening: I was finding evidence for my failure. Every time a runner came past me, it confirmed my worst fears: *I'm just not good enough, there is no point continuing. I'll be better off turning around and walking back to the start.*

It all seems silly now, but at the time it seemed like the truth.

If you feel like that, Ruth says there is a way through.

'The key thing there: recognise and manage your thought process. . . . you can do this by focusing on the external versus thoughts that are in your head. You need to find a strategy which will help you push through, and redirect your thoughts on things that will motivate you or get you back to your race plan. It can be something very simple, like, *Just relax*, or something more specific and technical aimed at that particular part of the race.'

On that day, the refocus for me was to think about my family, and that if I gave up and walked home, I would be letting them down. Over the years, different thoughts have worked in different races; sometimes even just focusing on moving my elbows in the run is enough to stop the negative thoughts.

Ruth Anderson explains: 'With thought control, you must learn to watch out for the early warning signs that your mind is not in the right state, that you are doubting your capacity to finish, not believing in your ability, and that is when you need to refocus on your race plan.'

The most surprising thing about learning to control your negative thoughts is that you start achieving results you wouldn't have hoped for, surpassing your expectations.

In those races where I have focused on the moment, concentrated on what I am doing, rather than letting invasive thoughts start dictating my actions, I have not only enjoyed the race far more but finished way ahead of where I had dared to imagine.

Four years on from my first race, it is still a battle of nerves for me, but it's one I am glad I am learning to fight.

CHAPTER 31

THE END OF THE ADVENTURE

'For the first time ever, nothing had gone wrong. I didn't lose a lens, fall off my bike, leave my helmet on back-to-front, or have to tie a shoelace.'

As I sit down to write this chapter, I find myself on what can only be described as a triathlon high, bursting full of endorphins and energy, even though my whole body is buzzing with exhaustion.

I have spent this past weekend racing, and the post-race euphoria has made me overexcitable, unable to sleep and already planning more races, while at the same time hobbling, a little bit achey and ravenously hungry.

This weekend I raced twice. The races were both frustrating and brilliant – and served to remind me why I love this sport and why I want to encourage others to take part, to join in and dare to try something they think is scary or impossible. (It doesn't have to be a triathlon!)

First up, on Saturday was a mixed relay supersprint in the grounds of the stunning Cholmondeley Castle in Cheshire. Of all the races I've entered so far, apart from my very first, this just might be my favourite.

The camaraderie in triathlon is unequalled. There is never a heavier dose of amiable support tinged with healthy competition than in a relay race.

My teammates were Lindsay Griffiths, a super-fit 33-year-old who used to serve in the Navy; 46-year-old Dave Morgan, who describes himself as a recreational Ironman; and 31-year-old Bradley Pollitt, who is a nervous swimmer but an incredibly strong cyclist and runner, and who would hopefully be our glory hunter for the last leg!

Mixed relay is a relatively new format added to the triathlon agenda. It is fast, furious and fantastic fun, and I particularly like the fact that men and women race together in the same teams.

There are two women and two men in the team. Everyone does each discipline – swim, bike, run – and then they pass the baton or tag their teammate so that the race can start all over again. The women go first and third. Right from the moment Lindsay asked me to be part of the team, I begged not to go first. On the day of the race, though, she had already competed in the morning, racing hard and winning her supersprint. My teammates therefore volunteered me to go first, so she could have an extra hour or so to recover.

The lake was warm and shallow, so we had to ease ourselves in rather than jump off the jetty. We had no time to acclimatise before we were off in a splash of yellow and green hats. With the pressure of the team's hopes as my motivation, I swam for my life and came out fourth, behind three girls who are part of the development squad for British Triathlon. I say 'girls' because they were the same ages as my daughters: 13 and 16.

The distances were short – only a 250-metre swim, a 5-kilometre bike and a 1.5 kilometre run – which means that it is over very quickly, and you cannot afford to lose a second or take a moment to catch your breath. I pushed as hard as I could but must have dropped two places on the bike and possibly another three on the run, leaving my team with work to do to get us back to where I had started, in fourth.

It wasn't long before transition resembled a teenager's bedroom with wetsuits, shoes and swimcaps strewn higgledy-piggledy all over the place. There was a constant shout of: 'Mind your backs, athlete coming through!' There was also plenty of friendly teasing about which team would be fastest – or the first to mess up.

By the time it got to the third or fourth leg, it was almost impossible to know where we were in the race. There was an endless huddle of triathletes in wetsuits, bouncing up and down nervously in the holding pen waiting for their runner to sprint towards them, make contact, and start their race.

We were all trying so hard that almost every runner collapsed in a heap on the ground when they finished. I nearly crashed through the barriers of the holding pen.

My teammates were impressively strong and fast. Between them, Dave and Lindsay made up all the places I had lost in the bike and the run, and we only had the youth development between us and a podium place.

It was now up to Brad to hold our position ahead of all the other age-groupers.

Brad hates the water but set off at a fast sprint to the jetty, neck and neck with the team who were competing for the very respectable fourth place. Even though he says he can't swim fast, he rushed back to transition at least 30 seconds ahead, and

I stood by him shouting encouragement (and trying not to put him off) and sent him on his way.

He was back from the bike in our fastest split of the day, and then in what seemed no time at all he was steaming down the finish line. We were just in time to greet him, and run under the finish banner together, hands held aloft.

We had finished fourth! Some people say that finishing fourth is the worst place, because you miss the podium by one slot. We didn't care. We had been beaten by the far superior, young, and hugely talented development team, all of them teenagers. Our motley crew were immensely proud to be a few minutes ahead of the rest of the age-groupers.

It is days like those that make me love my sport, surrounded by enthusiasts who have all worked hard to be there, and who now want to do their best and have fun.

That race was on Saturday. On Sunday, I raced again.

I don't think I have ever run the perfect race, but that day I came very close to it.

It wasn't easy, and it never will be. I didn't win, and there are a million things that I could do better. But it was great fun and reminded me why I have taken up sport late in life, and dedicated so much time and energy to it.

It was the Llandudno Sea Triathlon, on the North Wales coast, and it was a World Championship Sprint Distance Qualifier. I had never raced in a Sprint Distance Qualifier, as I am a better and more competitive endurance athlete over longer distances. A couple of days before the race, I did something I would never recommend doing. I checked the start list to see who was registered to qualify. It only served to intimidate me. In my age group, there were nine women registered to qualify, and to get in the team I would have to come at least fourth. The chances of that, given that sprint races are not my best distance, were very slim. But even if I didn't have much chance of qualifying, I still wanted to try my best.

As soon as I mention a sea swim, I imagine some people reading this might shudder. They would be right, too, particularly because this swim was in the Irish Sea – deep, dark, grey, murky, cold and choppy, with a current strong enough to carry you backwards. And yes, there were jellyfish, but not the nice floaty decorative kind that had hypnotised me in the docks in Liverpool; these were stingers. Thankfully, I didn't swim into one, but another competitor was not so lucky and got stung across her face. Bravely, she carried on.

It was drizzling when I racked my bike by the bus stop on the seafront, but I loved the whole day, right from the moment a group of triathletes from Manchester Tri Club tried to recruit me into their club. Their logic was that I work in Salford, just a hop, skip and a jump from Manchester, so I should join their club and leave Chester Tri Club.

Later, while listening to the race briefing over a speaker and wrapped up with a puffer jacket over my wetsuit to keep warm, I bumped into another lady in an older age group, flanked by her husband. They smiled through their shivers and told me it was all my fault that they were racing that day. Inspired by watching my adventures in triathlon on *BBC Breakfast* and after seeing me compete in the World Championships in Chicago, she took up the sport in her sixties. After only a year in triathlon, she had qualified for, and gone to, the World Championships in Cozumel – and she looked great on it.

Hearing stories like hers makes me proud and a bit emotional. If I can persuade one person to get up and try something they never thought possible, to get out there and get active, all my efforts and struggles are worth it.

Even I was intimidated by the start of the swim.

The bright yellow buoys were set up about 200 metres from the shoreline, which meant there was a considerable swim before the race even got underway. We had to wait, getting cold, on the beach for an additional agonising five minutes as the lifeboat brought back a man who had been struggling in the increasingly rough water. Seeing him being rescued did absolutely nothing to improve my nerves.

Health and Safety rules meant that before we were allowed to make our way towards the buoys, we had to get into the water and submerse ourselves for five minutes up to our necks, in order to acclimatise. I could only just spot the buoys in the distance, being thrown about by the swell. I talked nervously to my fellow athletes, teeth chattering, and laughed when others decided the best way to approach the challenge was to roar.

Yes, roar.

They did roar loudly, and it seemed very effective; everyone looked happier after they had done it.

We were all frozen and my hands were blue by the time we were told we could head away from the shoreline out to sea. It was a tough swim out there, as everyone jostled in the waves, trying to bag themselves a good position. When we got there, lining up between the buoys marking the start line was almost impossible: we were fighting the current in the deep water and being pushed backwards towards the pier. I had to do breaststroke just to keep still.

The waves, which had appeared small on the beach, felt about a metre high once I was swimming and being thrown up and down. Every time I took a breath, it was touch and go whether I also took a large gulp of seawater. When the race started the waves were so big I couldn't see where I was going, and I had to trust the women in front of me and hope they were going in the right direction. Soon I found myself on the wrong side of the marker buoys and being pushed inland, and I struggled to keep up. Once round the turnaround point, it all felt a little easier, and the waves began pushing me in the right direction. I started enjoying the swim in the final 100 metres as I made a beeline for the jetty.

Having struggled, I was determined I wouldn't be overtaken in transition and put in a burst of speed as I headed barefoot on the tarmac towards my bike. I totally nailed getting out of my wetsuit and seamlessly remembered to put my helmet and glasses on before touching my bike.

The cycle route was beautiful, but tough. It headed in a loop around Llandudno's Great Orme, a magnificent limestone headland that dominates the seaside town. There were a couple of hearty climbs at the start, followed by equally heart-stopping descents. Tricky switchbacks meant it was not a course for the faint-hearted. I know I am much faster on a descent than an ascent, so I held tight onto my handlebars, gritting my teeth while reaching speeds of more than 50 kilometres an hour.

I had come out of the swim first in my age group, and was then caught – as I thought I would be – by a couple of strong cyclists on the first loop around the town, putting me in third place. Doing my best to hold on, I put in maximum effort to keep ahead, because the run would be, as always, my weakest link.

I held my own until nearing the end of the second circuit. Then, pushing as hard as I could up a steep incline, I was passed by another woman on a bike matching mine, a Liv Envie. We laughed as we played tag for the final five kilometres. She would overtake me on the climbs, only for me to whizz past her on the descents. I shot into transition ahead of her, but even running in her cycle shoes, she was much faster than I was. She gleefully passed me with a cheery wave as I was still putting my shoes on for the run. That smile encapsulates for me why I think triathlon is such fun. There is no malice: we have all trained hard and are happy to be there, and if you are faster on the day, good on you! It will be well deserved, because it won't have come without hard work and effort.

I put everything I had into that run, keeping pace as best as I could with a younger runner, 20 metres in front of me. By my reckoning, I was probably at that stage fourth, and if I could hold it there, I would be in with a chance of the World Championships. The way my legs felt, heavy and leaden, I was right on the edge, with my heart rate near its max, but I wasn't going to give up. I focused on my elbows, thinking that if I could move them, my legs would move too.

The hill at the start of the Little Orme cost me more of my strength, but I was overjoyed to have made the turnaround with no one else catching me, and ran down letting my legs carry me as fast as I could. Every time I was overtaken I would hold my breath and hope it wasn't a woman in my age group. Every time it was a man it ignited a small glimmer of hope.

Back on to the Promenade with about half a kilometre to go, almost with the end in sight, it happened.

A lady with short red hair and wearing a black tri suit, who I had spotted racking her bike close to mine, now sprinted past me. It was as if she had just started out on a jog and wasn't on the verge of finishing a tough triathlon.

I had so nearly done it, so nearly made it, but there was nothing left in the tank, no turn of speed, no magic burst of acceleration. I nearly cried from pure frustration, but I didn't even have enough energy to do that. I tried to move faster, but didn't have it in me. I couldn't keep up with her, let alone beat her. By the time I had followed her into the finish, she had beaten me by 20 seconds. She was fourth and I was fifth. I had missed qualifying by 20 seconds. So near, but so far.

Holding on tight to the rail, I was nearly sick with exhaustion, leaning over and gasping for air as the volunteers put the medal around my neck. My new-found friends from Manchester Tri armed me with an alcohol-free beer, and as I got my breath back, I started to realise how nearly I had done it.

You can react to that sort of experience in different ways.

Initially, I was elated to have been good enough to have run her close, but also frustrated and annoyed with myself. *Just 20 seconds – how could I have let it come to just that? How infuriating! What could I have done?*

Just after the race, I bumped into my friend Andy Hamilton. He was commentating on the race that day, and is also a triathlon coach. He asked me a simple question.

'When she came past you, could you have sprinted for the finish?'

My answer was no.

'Did you do anything wrong in the race? Was there anything you could have done better?'

The honest answer was again no.

For the first time ever, nothing had gone wrong. I didn't lose a lens, fall off my bike, put my helmet on back to front or leave it on for the run, or have to tie a shoelace.

It had been my perfect race.

'You did your best, then. There is nothing more you could have done, and there is no shame in that. You should go home happy.'

And I did.

Happy about running my best race on the day. Happy about having taken part. Happy about being competitive. Happy about those euphoric moments when I was engrossed in the effort, focused on the fun, overrun by adrenaline, and engulfed by endorphins. Happy about daring to try.

It is the trying that makes me elated. To go to the World Championships again would be brilliant, but that is not why I compete. Chasing the glory isn't everything. I race, train and try hard because I love it.

It has been an amazing adventure . . .

CHAPTER 32

THE END OF THE ADVENTURE. WELL, NOT QUITE...

'Get a move on!'

David, my husband and most loyal supporter

I didn't expect to write this chapter.

But that's one of the many things I love about triathlon: very often things don't turn out quite as you imagine.

Six weeks after that fantastic weekend of triathlon, during which I had been training but with nothing like the intensity of getting ready for an important race, I had unexpected and exciting news.

An email from British Triathlon confirmed that my race results in Llandudno meant that I was in fact the proud owner of a Q for qualified. I had done it; I was back in the Great Britain team. I was made up.

The roll-down system had been at work and rolled down to my race time, which meant I had a place at the World Championships, this time in Rotterdam.

The race was only weeks away, so as well as ordering myself a snazzy new version of the Great Britain tri suit, I had to get back into serious training. I wanted to make sure that I didn't disgrace myself, or the team, by coming last.

The training was going brilliantly until I smashed my toe!

After a particularly chilly open-water swim in Manley Mere in Cheshire, with feet so freezing they had gone white, I jumped into my car without any shoes on, to warm up, and in my haste slammed the car door on my right foot. Even though my foot was numb from the cold, the pain was so excruciating I was nearly sick. What a total idiot!

I sat in agony, huddled in my car, and waited for the pain to subside. When it did, I sheepishly drove home, and didn't mention it to anybody; I knew my family would tell me how stupid I had been. Accustomed to a few triathlon bashes, I assumed I had just bruised it, and expected that the bruising would go away after a few days. It didn't. A week later, my poor little toe swelled up to twice its normal size – hot, red and angry. I hobbled around as best as I could and walked barefoot or in trainers all the time so that I didn't exacerbate the pain. The only exception was when I was sitting on the sofa for *Breakfast*, when I would wear my normal heels. I was pretty sure by now that it was much more than a bruise, it was broken. After googling what to do with a broken toe, it was perfectly obvious there was nothing that would offer a magical fix. All I could do was tape it up to my other toes, and wait for it to heal.

I was on countdown.

The World Championships in Rotterdam were three weeks away. I could still swim and cycle pretty well, but my walk was reduced to an ungainly hobble as I tried to keep pressure off my right foot. I was determined, though, that the small matter of a squashed toe wasn't going to stop me from trying to compete, so after a week of treatment with ibuprofen and ice, I went for a tentative run. Amazingly, it felt OK! For some reason, my toe didn't hurt nearly as much when I was running as when I was walking: it must have been down to the way I plant my foot. The trip was still on.

My next concern was the race itself.

One of my fellow athletes had emailed me a video of the bike course. There was a lot of discussion about its design among the age-groupers on Facebook. I watched the first 10 minutes and could see exactly what the fuss was all about: it was littered with dead turns, steep inclines, sharp bends, tram tracks, and benches and lamp posts in the middle of the path. This was described as a technical course, but looked downright dangerous. To make matters worse, the Sprint race was going to allow the use of the draft: tucking in close behind another cyclist, ensuring that you are carried along by their velocity and sheltered from the wind. It can save between 20 and 40 per cent of your energy, and enable you to cycle much faster. It is great fun when you get it right, but very challenging; you really have to concentrate and the slightest mistake can mean you crash into the person in front of you. We would be cycling in tight packs, at high speeds, inches away from each other's back wheel. And this would be only the second time I had raced with drafting permitted.

I had practised drafting with my friends as part of fun rides in Cheshire and group rides with Chester Triathlon Club, but never in a race situation. To feel more confident about drafting at race-pace on a tricky course, I needed to improve my bike handling skills. I spent an hour one afternoon in an empty car park, practising U-turns and perilous corners at speed, over and over again, until I felt more confident.

My arrival in Rotterdam was chaotic. After getting up at 3.30 a.m. to present *Breakfast*, I was feeling discombobulated as I was navigating my way through the airport some 18 hours later. Despite my lack of sleep, I thought I had everything under control, even my unwieldy bike box, until the moment I landed and started looking for my cash card to get some money out. It was nearly midnight when, in panic and desperation, I tipped out the contents of my bag on to the airport concourse – and confirmed not only had I misplaced my debit card, but that I had lost my entire wallet somewhere between buying a swimming hat and getting on the plane.

What a nightmare! It held my cash, my credit card and even my British Triathlon Federation card, without which I would not be allowed to race. I was distraught, annoyed with myself, and exhausted. Now it was too late to do much else beyond get to the hotel, check in, go to sleep and work out how to sort everything out when I felt less panicky.

To my amazement, the following morning, before I was even properly awake, I received a text from Emma Jones, one of the brilliant Assistant Editors on *Breakfast*. The news was fantastic: 'A woman at Manchester airport has emailed the programme, saying you left your purse in a shop and they are keeping it for you.'

Utterly brilliant!

And what are the chances? Someone had found it and handed it into a shop whose manager happened to be an avid *Breakfast* viewer. Opening it, they realised immediately who it belonged to and got in touch. Thanks to the power of *BBC Breakfast*, just a few short hours after losing my wallet, I knew it was safe – and they were sending it back to me.

The weather in Rotterdam was horrendous, with torrential rain lashing the streets and gusts of wind strong enough to lift 25-kilogram bike boxes. It felt ominously like the conditions in Chicago before my first World Championships. The turnout of Great Britain age-groupers was inspiring, though, with hundreds of us descending on the city to race. And we had a real treat in store.

The superstars of triathlon were competing the day before us, swimming in the same dock and on parts of the same course. In effect, we would be getting a masterclass in how to swim, bike and run – from the likes of Jonny Brownlee, Mario Mola, Javier Gómez, Flora Duffy, Jessica Learmonth and Jodie Stimpson, as well as the top paratriathletes, including the British Olympic gold medallist Andy Lewis.

It was the Grand Final of the ITU (International Triathlon Union), and I was reporting on it for the BBC's triathlon programme, which was live on BBC Two. What an incredible job to do: I had the privilege of talking about the sport I love with its most successful athletes and standing behind the finish line to watch them sprint up the blue carpet.

Not only did I get a close-up view of the elite races, I also got some top tips ahead of my own competition.

After interviewing two-time World Champion Flora Duffy, I asked for her advice on how to handle the tricky bike course. She told me to let my tyres down if it was going to be wet and slippery. This would give them more traction, and me more control over my bike, making me far less likely to crash on the cobbled surface. I did exactly as she said.

She wasn't the only one to give me some excellent advice. On the day of my race, I bumped into Andy Lewis, whom I had interviewed on the previous day, just moments after he won his second World Championship title. He very kindly took me to one side and explained how best to ride into and out of the sharp turns and difficult corners.

Jonny Brownlee told me it was a course for the brave triathlete, and these top tips did let me feel a little braver.

On race-day, I woke up feeling nervous and fidgety, as always – and had the added drama of waiting until the afternoon to start. There were hours ahead for my stomach to churn. The talk among fellow competitors tucking into breakfast was all about crashes. They were worried about a particularly dangerous section of the course, which involved a steep metal ramp on to a narrow bridge only just wider than my handlebars, with a ramp down the other side over a bump and a sharp left turn. It had only been set up overnight, so none of us who had recced the course in the days before had seen it. What's more, we already knew it was causing chaos.

Unaware of the danger ahead, the early waves of age-groupers had been streaming over the bridge, flying down the ramp and failing to make the turn, smashing into the barriers. I went to check it out, and by the time I got there the organisers had put a marshal with a flag slowing cyclists down before they hit the bridge. They had also moved the barriers. It was still very challenging, but it wasn't nearly as perilous.

Like the elites the day before, we had a split transition.

I had never competed in a triathlon with a transition like that, and it felt very odd to leave my trainers and a sports gel all on their own with no bike in T2 (Transition 2) before making my way over the elegant Erasmus Bridge, nicknamed 'The Swan', which connects the north and south of the city.

Everywhere I went, I was accompanied by other Great Britain age-groupers, all trying to navigate our way to T1 (Transition 1), which was on the other side of the Nieuwe Maas, the vast river that flows like an artery through the heart of Rotterdam.

My biggest concern was not to get cold before the swim started. I looked like a scarecrow when I turned up wearing my wetsuit, trainers, a fleece and a woolly hat to join David, Scarlett and Mia eating burgers and chips in the rustic Fenix Food

Factory near the start. It was too late for me to eat, or I would get a stitch, so I had a cup of coffee and watched enviously as a group of triathletes on a table beside us downed rounds of beer to celebrate finishing their races.

I was so delighted to be at the World Championships again, all I wanted to do was to finish the race safely, and enjoy it – and maybe, just maybe, improve on my 71st place finish in Chicago in 2015. As we lined up in pens before the start, I had a giggle with the women in my age group, laughing and taking pictures in our wetsuits and matching blue hats. Fun apart, the competition was tough and we had Australian Olympic silver medallist Michellie Jones in our wave, who also has a Paralympic gold medal to her name as the sighted guide for Australian Paralympian Katie Kelly at the Rio Games.

Unsurprisingly, it was Michellie who strode on to the blue pontoon first when we lined up for the swim start. I sat on the edge and watched the wave of women swimming in front of us. Right at the last minute, I got up and changed my position because I could see quite clearly that the women ahead of us were being pushed left by a current.

The klaxon sounded, and from that moment I loved the race.

The sun was out, and the water in the Rijnhaven, one of Rotterdam's oldest ports, felt warm and only a little bit choppy – in stark contrast to how it had been when I had been to the swim practice a couple of days before. Then, the waves had been huge, crashing over my head and making it hard to breathe without gulping mouthfuls of water.

As I turned around the first buoy, I followed the splashes of Michellie and the leaders streaming out ahead of me as guidance, and realised I was swimming side by side with one of my triathlon friends: Sam Gardiner. We met in Chicago, when she had stood on the side of that painful run course and cheered encouragement at me every time I passed her, shouting those epic words: 'When you hit the blue carpet, you are going to smile. And then you are going to look up and sprint to the finish line.'

I smiled at the memory, swimming stroke by stroke, like a synchronised swimmer, beside her. I knew the only place I could possibly beat her was the swim, and laughed as I scrambled to my feet two seconds ahead of her on the way into transition, where she overtook me.

The bike course was brilliant. Instead of being scary, it turned out to be mostly flat and in some sections very fast. I had done well on the swim, and as my fellow age-groupers came thundering past, I tried to pedal as hard as I could and stick to their back wheel and draft. They were all such strong cyclists, though, that it was tough to keep up.

I was so focused on staying safe and the speed of the course that I got a fright when I clattered over the metal bridge that had been worrying us all. The 20 kilometres sped by and I was swept towards the finish line in a large cluster of women in my age group. I was so relieved to have made it back safely that I made sure I came to a slow elegant halt before the dismount line. I stepped very carefully off my bike, then waved slightly hysterically to some *BBC Breakfast* fans shouting at me.

A very loud 'Get a move on!' from my husband, David, snapped me out of my mini-celebration, and I sprinted my way into transition. Running along beside me, as she had so many times before, was Scarlett, keeping me company on the other side of the fence. My shoes were by rack 49 and all I had to do to find them was to remember my age.

The 5-kilometre run in the late afternoon sunshine wound its way on gravel paths through trees bathed in autumnal hues in the city's Het Park. It was tough, as always, and my legs felt heavy, but this time I loved it. Only a short way to go, and then I could have a celebratory beer and a proper rest, and take my foot off the triathlon training treadmill.

The finish took me by surprise. It was an exhilarating sprint up the blue carpet, where I had seen the elites rack their bikes the day before, and the steep galleries on either side were packed with supporters. Buoyed by the noise of the crowds, I pushed as hard as I thought I could. With just 10 metres to go, out of the corner of my eye I glimpsed a Norwegian woman trying to catch me. With one last burst of speed I beat her by hundredths of a second over the finishing line, throwing my hands in the air with relief and exhilaration and falling into the arms of my teammates, who were celebrating their own successful races.

My two World Championship races couldn't have felt more different. Compared to that agonising run in the sweltering heat of Chicago, Rotterdam had been a blast from start to finish. I had wanted to have a safe and fun race, to end the season on a high – and I had done exactly that. The better news was that I had jumped 17 places – from 71st out of 77 competitors in Chicago, to 54th out of 77. If I hadn't faffed about and waved when I got off my bike, wasting at least 10 seconds, I could have come 50th.

I was ecstatic. What an incredible journey, to have come so far in such a short time. Even before I gave David, Mia and Scarlett a hug, I was already thinking, *I must do this again.*

Utter madness, of course!

But like any true triathlete, I know there is always the chance that next time I might just go even faster, and I know I won't be able to resist the temptation to race again.

THE FINISH LINE

It is now five years since I competed in my first triathlon. Since then, I have run, swam or cycled in more than 50 races, and I can remember every single one. There is so much I have loved about my endeavours – the training, the races, the friendships, the mistakes, the scary challenges – but it is only now, looking back, that I have started to realise how much it has changed me physically and mentally.

Physically, the difference is dramatic. I look different, I feel different. I am stronger, fitter and healthier. I sleep better, eat better, move better. Along with the scars from tumbles and falls along the way, the hours of training and racing are etched onto my physique, and this affects me 24 hours a day – from the moment the alarm goes off and I roll out of bed, to the way I sit on the sofa, walk to the shops, get up and make a cup of tea. My body is more robust and full of energy. I feel like I have found a magic formula.

Mentally it has also really helped, making me more resilient and determined.

I have learned it doesn't matter if I come last, if I fall, or if I fail. It is my resolve to get up and do it all over again that counts, the courage to dare to try and try some more. I know now that with effort and tenacity I can reach for goals that are seemingly beyond my grasp, and that with focus and determination the impossible becomes possible. That knowledge helps me in everything I do, it is not just relevant on race-day.

I am not only more resilient; I am also happier.

Each training swim, run or bike ride has lifted my mood, given me a break from fretful thoughts, made my worries seem smaller. I don't need to win, I don't even need to be in a competition to feel the benefits of exercise; they are with me every minute of every day and have become part of my personality.

We talk so much on *BBC Breakfast* of mental and physical health and what can be done to help people. For me, the answer has been triathlon. It is not for everyone, but I would love to persuade you to put on a pair of trainers, sign up for a sponsored swim, set out on a 20-kilometre bike ride. Whatever you choose, just dare to try. See where your journey takes you. And, if you see me in the race, give me a wave on your way past!

And when you get to the finish line of your own challenge, remember: it isn't really the finish, it's the start of the next adventure (and I'm already planning mine!)

Louise x

USEFUL RESOURCES

Inspired to start your own sporting adventure? Trust me, if I can do it I have no doubt you can too. Check out these useful contacts and with any luck, we will be competing alongside one another in the not too distant future.

Women in Sport's mission is to empower women and girls through sport and the sport sector, visit www.womeninsport.org/our-mission/

If fear of being judged on appearance or performance is holding you back from trying triathlon (or any other sport), visit www.thisgirlcan.co.uk

To find out more about triathlon in Great Britain, visit www.britishtriathlon.org

To join the 'Women for Tri' community, visit www.womenfortri.com/

First time out? To find a 'beginner' triathlon in your area, and advice on how to prepare for it, visit www.active.com/triathlon/beginner

For low-cost, fun and short-distance triathlons, perfect for newcomers to the sport, visit www.gotri.org

For information on local running, cycling and triathlon clubs, visit www.timeoutdoors.com/clubs

For information on wild swimming and a calendar of events in the UK and beyond, visit www.outdoorswimmingsociety.com

For additional information about open-water swimming, finding a safe venue or an approved event, visit www.sh2out.org

For advice on all aspects of cycling, visit www.britishcycling.org.uk

To hone your skills in the cycling time trial element of triathlon, visit the National Governing Body for Cycling Time Trials' website: www.cyclingtimetrials.org.uk

To get into 'extreme' triathlon with Ironman, visit www.eu.ironman.com/

RECORDS

Since I started competitive sport again in 2012 I have done dozens of different races. These are the results from the events that I have talked about at length in this book.

Date	Race	Swim distance	Swim time	T1	Bike distance	Bike time	T2	Run distance	Run time	Total	Place (age-group)	Place (female)
21.07.13	Deva Divas	750m	14.02	0.56	25k	52.32	1	5k	26.44	1.34.59	8/57	43/273
Sep 2013	Bridge to Bridge Swim	5k	1.43.00									1st wetsuit
21.09.13	Brownlee Super Sprint	400m	6.58	2.2	10k	25.24	1.1	2.5	14.17	49.29	4/49	
May 2014	Manchester 10k							10k	56.19			
June 2014	Milligan Bike Ride				500k (300 miles)	3 days						
Sep 2014	Brownlee Tri North	750m	14.21	1.43	26k	1.04.06	1.17	5.5k	32.32	1.53.59	4/15	25/144
Mar 2015	Dyfi Dash (Machynlleth)	400m	7.28	3.15	20k	40.33	0.22	5k	36.13	1.27.54	4	33/123
19.04.15	Chirk Tri	400m	6.57	1.23	25k	48.15	0.56	5k	25.37	1.23.10	9/27	36/123
10.05.15	Great Manchester Run							10k	51.42			
30.05.15	Dee Mile	2k	29.38								14/111	60/300
14.06.15	Deva Triathlon Chester	1,500m	23.42	1.40	40k	1.18.41	1.12	10k	52.46	2.38.03	20/32	128/256
20.06.15	Dambuster Tri Ripon	1,500m	25.22	1.23	40k	1.27.47	1.10	10k	53.11	2.48.55	7	95
26.07.15	Liverpool Sprint Tri	750m	12.25	3.51	20k	40.47	3.21	5k	26.05	1.26.29	1/11	14/96
19.09.15	World Championships Chicago	750m	11.28	4.19	37k	1.12.25	3.36	10k	1.05.07	2.36.53	71/78	
29.05.16	European Championships Lisbon	1,500m	25.02	1.31	40k	1.28.03	1.16	10k	54.19	2.50.13	32/35	
14.09.16	Serpentine Swim	1 mile	25.49								5	31
06.11.16	New York City Marathon							26.2 miles	5.51.46			
17.09.17	World Championships Rotterdam	750m	12.51	5.43	20k	42.07	2.36	5k	26.34	1.29.48	54/77	

ACKNOWLEDGEMENTS

First, thanks go to the brilliant and inspired Nadia Dahabiyeh from *BBC Breakfast* for coming up with the Velodrome Challenge and changing my life for ever.

Thanks to Adam Bullimore, *BBC Breakfast* editor, and to all my wonderful colleagues who work on the programme, for putting up with my endless stories, bumps and bruises.

Thanks to Chester Tri Club for their advice, friendship and coaching and for organising the best races. Thanks especially to the running coaches who have never made me feel like a fool.

Thanks to Global Bike, Alf Jones Cycles, Sixty Nine Cycles and Liv Cycling for helping me with all my bike issues, big or small, and to Yonda Sports wetsuits.

A huge thank you to Claire Sutcliffe, my coach, who has always believed in me and supported every madcap idea with enthusiasm and clear guidance. Without her, I would never have made it into the GB Team.

Thanks to all the GB age-group athletes for making me feel included and part of the team and for their support and encouragement every step of the way, especially on the agonising runs at the end of the races.

Special thanks to the strong and inspiring women I compete with in my age group, and who are now my friends: Mo McDowall, Ceri Cook, Melanie Betts, Sam Gardiner and Sharon Plested.

Thanks to the race official who picked me up off the tarmac in Liverpool and sent me on my way to my first age-group win and to all the supporters who have cheered me on in a race. I heard every one of you, and you each made a difference.

Thanks to all the *BBC Breakfast* viewers who over the years have sent me messages of support for my endeavours, and especially those who contacted me on that stormy night before the World Championships in Chicago and inspired me to carry on.

Thank you to the Team GB triathletes Non Stanford, Vicky Holland, Jodie Stimpson and Alistair and Jonathan Brownlee for their support and for humouring my attempts to mimic their footsteps.

Thanks to BBC Sport's Ron Chakraborty and Sarah Richardson for seeing my passion and letting me talk about the sport I love, presenting the BBC's triathlon coverage.

And finally, thank you to Matthew Lowing at Bloomsbury for tracking me down and asking me to write this book and for his humour, gentle guidance and encouragement along the way.

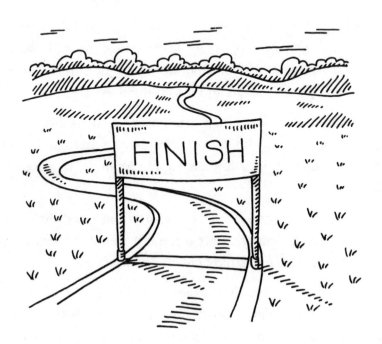